SHATTERING CULTURE

SHATTERING CULTURE

AMERICAN MEDICINE RESPONDS TO CULTURAL DIVERSITY

MARY-JO DELVECCHIO GOOD,
SARAH S. WILLEN, SETH DONAL HANNAH,
KEN VICKERY, AND LAWRENCE TAESENG PARK

EDITORS

Russell Sage Foundation • New York

The Russell Sage Foundation

The Russell Sage Foundation, one of the oldest of America's general purpose foundations, was established in 1907 by Mrs. Margaret Olivia Sage for "the improvement of social and living conditions in the United States." The Foundation seeks to fulfill this mandate by fostering the development and dissemination of knowledge about the country's political, social, and economic problems. While the Foundation endeavors to assure the accuracy and objectivity of each book it publishes, the conclusions and interpretations in Russell Sage Foundation publications are those of the authors and not of the Foundation, its Trustees, or its staff. Publication by Russell Sage, therefore, does not imply Foundation endorsement.

Library of Congress Cataloging-in-Publication Data

Shattering culture : American medicine responds to cultural diversity / Mary-Jo DelVecchio Good . . . [et al.], editors.
   p. cm.
  Includes bibliographical references and index.
  ISBN 978-0-87154-060-7 (pbk. : alk. paper)—ISBN 978-1-61044-752-2 (ebook)
1. Medical care—United States. 2. Cultural pluralism. I. Good, Mary-Jo DelVecchio.
  RA410.53.S52 2011
  362.10973—dc23

2011022410

Text design by Suzanne Nichols.

RUSSELL SAGE FOUNDATION
112 East 64th Street, New York, New York 10065
10 9 8 7 6 5 4 3 2 1

We dedicate this book to Byron Good,
Sebastian Wogenstein, Shelly Hannah,
Avery Rose Hannah, Jennifer Park, and Carol Sun.

Contents

About the Authors

Mary-Jo DelVecchio Good is professor of social medicine at Harvard Medical School and teaches in the Department of Sociology at Harvard University, in addition to being a faculty affiliate of the Asia Center, the Center for Middle Eastern Studies, and the Weatherhead Center for International Affairs.

Sarah S. Willen is assistant professor of anthropology at the University of Connecticut.

Seth Donal Hannah is lecturer on sociology at Harvard University.

Ken Vickery is director of external fellowships at the University of Illinois, Urbana-Champaign.

Lawrence Taeseng Park is assistant professor of psychiatry at Massachusetts General Hospital.

Antonio Bullon is assistant professor of psychiatry, director of neuropsychiatry education, and director of the Latino Mental Health Service at the Beth Israel Deaconess Medical Center.

Joseph D. Calabrese is lecturer in medical anthropology at University College, London.

Elizabeth Carpenter-Song is assistant professor in the Department of Community and Family Medicine and Anthropology at Dartmouth College.

Sadeq Rahimi is assistant professor of medical anthropology at the University of Saskatchewan.

Lisa Stevenson is assistant professor of anthropology at McGill University.

Marina Yaroshenko is staff psychiatrist at Massachusetts General Hospital.

Acknowledgments

In the spring of 2001, I was invited by Brian Smedley, the study director for the Institute of Medicine's (IOM) Group on Racial and Ethnic Disparities, to consider the question of how well-meaning physicians could provide inequitable care to minority and nonminority patients. After initial literature reviews and conversations with medical colleagues, most notably Guiseppe Raviola, Elizabeth Herskovits, and Anne Becker, I reframed the committee's study question from a psychological one attuned to personal bias to a social one attuned to culture to ask how the culture of medicine—including the training of medical students and residents and the organization and delivery of health care—affects patient treatment in such a way as to produce disparities in therapeutic action and the quality of care. I asked my HMS colleagues Anne Becker and Byron Good and my graduate student Cara James to join me in responding to the IOM request. Drawing on our research on medical education and the comparative cultures of medicine and psychiatry, I focused our contribution on what medicine cares about: time and efficiency, hierarchies of valued knowledge dominated by the biomedical sciences, and appreciation for patients who willingly enter the world of medicine and who do not have socially complex problems (Good 1994; 1995). In reviewing disparities in mental health care, we looked to aspects of psychiatric practice that might lead to disparities in diagnosis and treatment, such as aversive racism (Dovidio and Gaertner 2004; Good et al. 2003), and major efforts of the past several decades in building medical education and training in cultural competence. "The Culture of Medicine and Racial, Ethnic, and Class Disparities in Healthcare" (Good et al. 2003) served the committee as a background paper used in writing the report and was included in the publication *Unequal Treatment: Confronting Racial and Ethnic Disparities in Healthcare* (Smedley, Stith, and Nelson 2003).

Writing "The Culture of Medicine and Racial, Ethnic and Class Disparities in Healthcare" in the summer of 2001 sparked ideas for a new research agenda, which I presented at a Russell Sage Foundation conference on medical anthropology and culture contact, held on October 12, 2001, a grave time for New York City and the United States. This RSF conference and the work I did for IOM launched a course of study and exploration on how culture matters in American medicine. In 2002–2003 I had the good fortune to spend a year as a visiting scholar at Russell Sage Foundation, and concomitantly received a small presidential grant to conduct pilot research on the culture of medicine and disparities in treatment in the Boston area (2002–2004). In 2005, Eric Wanner and Jitka Maleckova encouraged me to design a broader project, eventually funding "How Does Culture Make a Difference in American Health Care? American Health at the Interface of Ethnicity/Race and Citizenship" (2006–2009). Thus, I am most grateful to the Russell Sage Foundation and its president Eric Wanner for this near decade-long support, to RSF's program officers, Stephanie Platt and Jitka Maleckova, to the foundation's trustees, who were enthusiastic about research on the culture of medicine, especially Melvin Konner and Christine Castle, to Louise Lamphere from the Culture Contact group, to Suzanne Nichols for her wise shepherding through the publication process, and to April Rondeau for her excellent work during the copyediting and proofing stages. The RSF-funded research project supported the empirical studies at the core of the chapters of *Shattering Culture*.

I greatly appreciate the postdoctoral and predoctoral fellows at the Department of Social Medicine, Harvard Medical School, who contributed to the project on culture and medicine at various stages of the research from research design to field studies, each bringing unique contributions and great creativity and energy to the many tasks involved in such an enormous endeavor. NIMH postdoctoral fellows who participated included: Lawrence T. Park, a psychiatrist and anthropologist who became site principal investigator at a large healthcare institution and its satellites, where we carried out research, and who was deeply engaged in research design; anthropologists Lisa M. Stevenson, Sarah S. Willen, Elizabeth Carpenter-Song, Joseph Calabrese, and Ken Vickery, who participated in various ways from design to field observations, interviewing, and analysis; predoctoral fellow and sociologist Seth Donal Hannah, who was engaged in all phases of the research; and psychiatrist Marina Yaroshenko, who was engaged in design, interviewing, and smoothing the way for clinical observations and interviews of other fellows. Sadeq Rahimi, a Canadian Research Council postdoctoral fellow in culture and psychiatry, was involved from project design through field interviews. In addition to our fellows, psychiatrist Antonio Bullon led the research at one site as clinical site PI and interviewer and researcher. All participated in data analysis and in contributing to the chapters in this book. Our fellows were superbly supported by the excellent work of our scientific staff and project researchers/managers, Matt Lakoma and Elisa Poorman (Elisa interviewed many clinicians, interpreters, and patients and translated and conducted interviews in Spanish and transcribed), and by Seth Hannah in his guise as a project manager, field researcher, and chief data analyst. My staff assistants, Anna Lisa Silva and Laura French Delano, and many Harvard College students transcribed interviews and provided helpful analytic notes and commentary. These included Miki Cohen Moskowitz, who also conducted interviews with Elisa Poorman, and Pearl Houghteling, Lizzy Majzoub, Nicole Piedra, Rachel Reardon, Lisa Weiss, Veronica Cordova, Aparna Chatterjee, and R. Santos. We thank Debra Keaney for smoothly and skillfully managing our grant finances.

Anthropological and ethnographic research in psychiatric clinical and hospital settings is extremely difficult, requiring exceptional efforts by colleagues not directly engaged in the research to smooth the way for ethnographers to carry out formal interviews as well as to observe and engage in conversations. We, the editors and authors, are most grateful for the exceptional contributions of all our medical colleagues, in particular our site PIs. Dr. Anne Becker, psychiatrist, provided insightful consultations on our research design and assumed the position of site PI when Dr. Park left Boston for the FDA; Dr. Alastair Donald, site PI at a health-care institution, facilitated observations in psychiatric units and interviews with patients and mental health workers. We also thank those many psychiatrists and hospital and clinic directors who made our research possible by approving our project and introducing it to clinical staff, including Jonathan Worth, Jennifer Lafayette, Mary-Lyons Hunter, Hodan Mohammed, Tony Raynes, Stuart Carter, Joseph Dipietro, Maria Stacey, Mark Schecter, David Geltman, Nina Calabrezze, Jonathan Borus, and Shelonda Scott Hannah. We greatly appreciate the generosity of the many psychiatrists, residents, clinicians, chaplains, medical educators, interpreters, health-care staff, and patients who participated in the study, engaged in conversations, and were willing to give their time to be interviewed and to share their views.

Shattering Culture emerged through an ongoing conversation of over two decades on medical anthropology, culture, and psychiatry generated in the Friday Morning seminars sponsored by our Harvard Training Program in Culture and Mental Health Services Research, funded by the National Institutes of Mental Health, and directed by Byron Good, Arthur Kleinman, and Mary-Jo DelVecchio Good. Special seminar sessions and featured workshops ranged across topics as diverse as cross-cultural research and therapeutics, to understanding and treating refugees and immigrants, to designing clinics to redress disparities and inequalities in mental health care for ethnic, racial, or linguistic minorities. We often asked how culture—of patients or of medicine and psychiatry—makes a difference in mental health care. Seminars and special workshops held between 2006 and 2008 featured new research on medicine and psychiatry's responses to immigration and increasing cultural diversity. Many of our invited speakers were deeply engaged in thinking about how culture matters in health policies to reduce disparities and inequalities and to improve psychiatric understanding and care by attending to the cultural aspects of patients and of care. We greatly appreciate the National Institute of Mental Health for twenty-four years of support for the Research Training Program in Culture and Mental Health Services (5 T32 MH 18006), and for support for the fellows who participated in this research. We are truly amazed by and grateful for the generosity of our intellectual community who energized our research, including regular seminar participants as well as featured visitors, many of whom were formerly fellows. Thus the editors wish to thank all who offered their expertise, insights, and advice and who made helpful commentaries on seminar and workshop presentations which evolved into the chapters in *Shattering Culture*. These include Janis Jenkins, Tom Csordas, Antonio Bullon, Doris Chang, Michael M. J. Fischer, Atwood Gaines, Linda Garro, Peter Guarnaccia, Devon Hinton, Ladson Hinton, Jean Jackson, Erica James, Arthur Kleinman, Robert LeVine, Roberto Lewis-Fernandez, Amaro Laria, Cheryl Mattingly, Michael and Michelle Nathan, Henry Grunebaum, and Amelie Rorty. We also thank the many graduate students in medical anthropology who brought fresh perspectives and joy to our seminars, including Felicity Aulino, Adia Benton, Jesse Grayman, Sharon Abramowitz, and Michelle Levine. Ronald Angel, Philippe Bourgois, Louise Lamphere, Ken Fox, Steve Lopez, and William Vega as well as many colleagues previously mentioned also participated in a workshop at RSF in February 2003 which engaged the nascent ideas that led to the research and this book. We also wish to thank RSF's two anonymous reviewers whose suggestions improved the quality of the book once it was in draft form.

I offer a special acknowledgment to Janis Jenkins, my dear colleague and friend, who was with me when we first conceptualized this research, advised us throughout from design to publication with tough mindedness and intellectual generosity. And finally, through more than forty years of our marriage, Byron and I have been collaborators in research and in writing projects. Although his name does not appear on any of these essays, his spirit is fully present. Byron was engaged in energizing and developing ideas that led to the research, and delighted as we moved toward analysis. As ever, his gift of love to us all is through kindly offered suggestions and recommendations in response to what we write, and in the minutiae of his superb copyediting.

Mary-Jo DelVecchio Good
Cambridge, Massachusetts
July 2011

References

Good, Byron. 1994. *Medicine, Rationality, and Experience: An Anthropological Perspective,* vol. 1990. Cambridge and New York: Cambridge University Press.

Good, Mary-Jo DelVecchio. 1995. *American Medicine, the Quest for Competence.* Berkeley: University of California Press.

Dovidio, John F., and Samuel L. Gaertner. 2004. "Aversive Racism." *Advances in Experimental Psychology* 36(1): 1–52.

Good, Mary-Jo DelVecchio, Cara James, Byron J. Good, Anne E. Becker. 2003. "The Culture of Medicine and Racial, Ethnic, and Class Disparities in Healthcare." In *Unequal Treatment: Confronting Racial and Ethnic Disparities in Healthcare,* edited by Brian D. Smedley, Adrienne Y. Stith, and Alan R. Nelson. Washington, D.C.: National Academies Press.

Smedley, Brian D., Adrienne Y. Stith, and Alan R. Nelson. 2003. *Unequal Treatment: Confronting Racial and Ethnic Disparities in Healthcare.* Washington, D.C.: National Academies Press.

Chapter 1

Shattering Culture: An Introduction

MARY-JO DELVECCHIO GOOD WITH
SETH DONAL HANNAH AND SARAH S. WILLEN

H OW DOES culture matter in American medicine and health care? This query motivated the ethnographic studies of health-care institutions and psychiatric clinics that are the heart of this volume.

Why Attend to Culture in Medicine and Health Care Now?

For many decades, American medicine and its institutions of patient care have attended to the cultural distinctiveness of patients and carried out missions to redress inequalities in access to medical services for the poor, for ethnic and racial minorities, and for new immigrants and refugees.[1] However, despite years of effort to institutionalize culturally sensitive and competent care and to reach out to serve and provide equitable care to minority patients, two highly consequential federal policy studies, *Mental Health: Culture, Race, and Ethnicity* and *Unequal Treatment*, released in 2001 and 2002–2003, respectively, reported persistent inequalities and disparities in treatment by culture, race, and ethnicity over a wide range of psychiatric and medical specialties (Smedley, Stith, and Nelson 2003; Surgeon General 2001). Studies funded by the National Institutes of Health over the past two decades also found that unequal medical and psychiatric treatment cannot be explained by differences in access or by individual patient characteristics alone, thereby leading researchers and

1

policymakers to seek explanations in subtle and complex psychological, social, and cultural processes in interactions between patients and their doctors and health-care institutions. The public discussions generated by these two policy discussions on "culture counts" and "unequal treatment" remain profoundly vibrant and relevant in health policy and medical circles today.

This book reports on findings from a study carried out in Greater Boston, in which we explored the role of culture in contemporary worlds of medicine and psychiatry as practiced in environments of increasingly complex cultural and demographic diversity. With the publication of these reports, the concept of culture came to have a newfound caché in American medicine in the twenty-first century. The social milieu generating this dynamism in the meaning and importance of culture is the dramatic transformation in the demographic landscape of American society.[2] The new immigration over the past several decades has intensified American cultural diversity and increased complex formulations of racial and ethnic identities (Lee and Bean 2010). We define this as the emergence of cultural environments of hyperdiversity (see chapter 2, this volume).

The chapters in this book discuss the various ways culture is used and given meaning in psychiatry and mental health care in clinical settings in Greater Boston. Our research documented how ideas about culture, ethnicity, immigration, diversity, disparities, and inequalities are shaped in and by American medicine and its institutions of patient care, research and training, and health policy, thereby influencing clinical ideologies, forming clinical practices, and generating programs to deliver quality care that is regarded as culturally appropriate, sensitive, or competent. We sought to understand the roles and meanings of culture from the perspective of clinicians and health-care staff who treat patients from diverse cultural backgrounds and who find culture relevant in their daily clinical work, asking them to reflect not only on patient culture but also on the culture of psychiatry and medicine and of their clinics—in other words, organizational culture.

We framed our research with two overarching queries: How does American medicine respond to cultural diversity? Does culture make a difference in American health care and in mental health care? We began the research with three broad issues in mind.[3] First, we wondered about the extent to which notions of ethnicity and culture, popular in the 1960s when community clinics were being established as part of the Great Society agenda,[4] remain present in the way doctors and clinics use culture and think about how culture counts; the extent to which the language of cultural competence in contemporary medicine relies on ideas of an earlier era, of coherent ethnic communities sharing coherent cultures; and whether these older models of ethnicity are still regarded as useful guides for clinicians and those who organize care in today's culturally diverse medical settings. Second, we wondered about the extent to which ideas of race, ethnicity, and culture are shaped by changing demographics and the new immigration (for a review, see Suárez-Orozco, Suárez-Orozco, and Qin 2005 and Kasinitz et al. 2008), and whether newer ideas of culture that no longer assume coherent systems of meaning and experience have found their way into the discourses, practices, and policies of American medicine and psychiatry. Third, and most fundamental to our research, we consider how the culture of medicine and in particular the culture of psychiatry adapt and respond to these changes and how broad symbolic systems that support American medicine and its subspecialties interact with the dynamic and changing meanings of ethnicity, race, and culture that have evolved over the past two decades.

The terms *shattering culture* and *cultural environments of hyperdiversity* (or, simply, *hyperdiversity*), from which we draw our title, emerged directly from our ethnographic investigations and observations. Hyperdiversity, as Seth Hannah discusses in chapter 2, identifies our nation's dynamic population transition to a complex and mosaic-like mix of national origin, ethnicity, race, immigration status and nativity. *Shattering Culture,* our title, popped out as we analyzed our interviews and observations. The title identifies the uncertainty that arises in these cultural environments of hyperdiversity in which broad identity-based indicators of cultural difference are often too blunt to capture current social and individual identities. The new immigration and the new ethnic-racial mix in younger generations of Americans and immigrants have shattered bounded communities and the cultural meanings of the old social categories of ethnicity and race, as cultural identities have increasingly become more complex, dynamic, fluid, and evolving.[5] Census categories of the race and ethnicity pentad are gradually breaking apart in a dynamic and ever-evolving fashion (Asian, black, Hispanic, Native American and Pacific Islander, and white, with mixed race added in this decade). Thus the certainty of these official cultural categories, the result of so much health and other government policy research, is shattered (Prewitt 2005, 2009; Saulny 2011).

The politically important cultural categories of race and ethnicity have been fundamental to promoting civil rights, to assessing inequalities and disparities "in health, education, housing, and civil rights protection, and to identifying underrepresented minorities" (Saulny 2011, A1). And yet they now seem, at least in popular culture, to be social labels and analytic categories of another era and to have diminished political potency and meaning (CDC 2011).[6] Shattering culture also names efforts of clinicians and support staff who attend to emergent and contextually dependent patterns of social categorization and ways individuals appropriate and use cultural difference. For example, language, income, and insurance status were often considered as important cultural categories that rivaled or exceeded race and ethnicity. In using the term *shattering culture,* we do not intend to discard culture as a concept with which to think and make sense of the world of medicine and of social life, but rather to note that the certainty about the value of older cultural categories of race and ethnicity, used often in establishing social policies for equality and the common good, is shattered.

In the following sections of this chapter, we discuss psychiatry's import for understanding the meanings and uses of culture in medicine and responses to cultural diversity today, and follow with an exploration of the issues framed by, and in conversation with, the two highly significant national health policy discussions of this century—culture counts in mental health care and unequal treatment and disparities in healthcare. We present a discussion of the demographic landscape of Boston and its uniqueness and a description of our research design, clinical sites, and the sample characteristics of our participants. We conclude with a brief preview of the chapters.

Anthropology in Psychiatric Clinical Settings

Why psychiatry? Culture has long been a fundamental analytic category with political and policy caché in psychiatry and mental health services, as well as among academic research communities. Questions about whether mental illnesses vary across cultures, and about how to adapt psychiatric services—including diagnosis, therapeutics, and the organization of care—for the various needs of distinctive cultures and subcultures, have been central issues of concern for nearly the whole of modern psychiatry (see Anderson, Jenson, and Keller 2011; Kleinman and Good 1986). Historically rooted in engagements with cultures around the globe since colonial eras (Pols 2011; Anderson, Jenson, and Keller 2011; Good and Good 2010; Jenkins and Barrett 2004), psychiatry has held a fascination for cultural difference in how mental illness is expressed, experienced, and understood (Good and Good 2010).

Thus, psychiatry today is the ideal medical specialty to study where culture counts, what culture means, and how disparities and inequalities in treatment by race and ethnicity are linked to issues of culture as they are debated and discussed. It is the field of medicine where the meaning of culture is most seriously and frequently considered and assessed; where culture is used as a clinical frame and a valuable concept for teaching residents how to create trusting relationships with patients (Kleinman, Eisenberg, and Good 1978); where universalism and cultural specificity are common in discourses on patient care, therapeutics, and diagnostics; and where cultural systems of meaning and experience are relevant for clinicians as much as for their patients (Good and Good 1980). Psychiatry is the medical discipline most often charged with teaching cultural competence and cultural sensitivity to medical students, residents, and other clinical trainees, and the specialty most concerned with language barriers and clinician-patient matching (Willen, Bullon, and Good 2010; chapters 3 and 5, this volume). In addition, psychiatrists are most frequently turned to by physicians from other specialties for cultural consultations.[7]

Psychiatry is also the medical specialty that reflects most deeply on its own internal variety and diversity of professional cultures, such as acknowledging the tension between universalism and cultural specificity, as well as the competition among psychodynamic, cultural, biological, neuroscience, and—most recently—genetic approaches to making sense of mental illness, designing therapeutics, and understanding humankind (Luhrmann 2000; Jenkins 2011; Lewis-Fernandez, personal correspondence, March 2011). For example, today's leading cultural psychiatrists[8] are shaping cultural ideologies for ethnic specific clinics, creating cultures of clinical practice oriented toward culturally diverse patient populations served, and actively undertaking cross cultural research. They are creating one dimension of psychiatry's culture of the twenty-first century by developing new diagnostic definitions and illustrative cases where patient culture matters in treatment, for the American Psychiatric Association's Diagnostic and Statistical Manual (DSM) 5.0.[9] They also debate the merits of universalism and cultural specificity in patient care, exploring ways to balance these two impulses in American psychiatry "that allow one to transcend difference and seek affinities across cultural boundaries."[10] Thus the drive toward encompassing cultural particularism into universalism (a culturally constructed notion as well) at the heart of today's cultural psychiatry is not surprising. As Roberto Lewis-Fernandez, a leading cultural psychiatrist speaking about the work of the DSM 5.0[11] working group on culture says, "I am not anti-universalism, but for a more informed universalism."

Similar to many other fields in medicine, psychiatry is also under stress from current financial constraints and chaotic coverage and payment plans, as well as from an explosion in documentation practices and technological modes of regulation and oversight (see chapters 10 and 11, this volume). Thus for those interested in how medicine is responding to cultural diversity today, psychiatry is a field that is good to think with.

Culture Counts and Unequal Treatment

Psychiatry has long been concerned with cultural differences in access and use of mental health services and in treatment outcomes. Beginning in the 1960s, research began to show differences in access to care, treatment quality, and outcomes for racial and ethnic minorities in the United States, leading to debates among psychiatrists, policymakers, and other activists about the potential explanations for these troubling differences

(Sue 1977). Some took the particularistic position that culture counts, arguing that cultural barriers to treatment caused unequal outcomes. They viewed the experience and expression of mental illness as fundamentally different across diverse racial and ethnic groups and argued these differences must be taken into account to provide effective and equitable treatment for all (Sue 1998; Satcher 2001; Chang 2003). Researchers also proposed that inferior care could be caused by racism or bias on the part of individual providers or the system itself (Smedley, Stith, and Nelson 2003). Others looked to more universalistic explanations, that racial and ethnic differences in access to psychiatric care, quality of care, and treatment outcomes are due to universal aspects of mental illness, and that individual characteristics such as social class, poverty, and lifestyle choices are disproportionately present in different groups (Chang 2003).

These concerns with differences in mental health care by race and ethnicity of over thirty years ago were motivated in part by the identity politics of the 1960s and the social movements promoting equality for racial and ethnic groups in the United States, defined by the U.S. Census pentad, as white, African American, Asian, Hispanic/Latino, and Native American and Pacific Islanders (Hannah 2011). They were also motivated by a global deinstitutionalization movement to close the mental hospitals and asylums and replace them with community mental health and outpatient services. These two movements transformed American psychiatric treatment from long-term hospitalization or asylum care (Goffman 1961) to short-term stays, outpatient medication, and culturally sensitive and tailored treatment at many community mental health centers.[12] Thus the politics of designing culturally appropriate care radically changed with the changes in treatment modalities and settings, and culture, race, and ethnicity became politically significant to building services designed to serve minority populations.

Themes from this earlier era continue to be central today in reports on culture counts and unequal treatment reflecting a renewed concern about the burden of mental illness for racial and ethnic minorities and inequalities in treatment. Many of the same academics who were advocates for minority mental health in the 1960s and 1970s participated in the production of these twenty-first century reports and remain leading advocates today. In 1999, the Surgeon General released a mental health report that identified the disease burden of mental illness and access to mental health care as an area of growing concern for the United States, but framed the issue in universal terms, neglecting to report on differences in prevalence, treatment, and care for racial and ethnic minorities. Academic experts in minority mental health, often members of the groups they study, regarded the exclusion of analyses by culture, race, and ethnicity as deplorable, as did the federal employees most engaged in policies promoting mental health care for ethnic and racial minorities (see Chang, Good, and Good

2003). They successfully lobbied for a new consensus report, *Mental Health: Culture, Race, and Ethnicity, A Supplement to the Surgeon General's Report on Mental Health* (Surgeon General 2001), which highlighted the importance of race and ethnicity, declaring that culture counts. They documented ways culture counts in mental health care and health policy through empirical studies, identifying by culture, race, and ethnicity the unequal burden of mental illness, unequal use and access to treatment, and disparities and inequalities in diagnosis, medication, therapeutics and quality of care (Chang et al. 2003; Chang 2003; Surgeon General 2001). "Culture Counts" fast became a rallying cry for those promoting programs for minority mental health. The phrase resonates well with the long tradition of using culture as a fundamental albeit diffuse analytic category in psychiatry, justifying attention to cultural variation in the experience and expression of illness and legitimizing investment in culturally tailored mental health services and culturally competent care.[13]

Nonetheless, a tension between impulses to privilege cultural distinctiveness versus universal commonalities is common as well in research that does attend to minority mental health and analytic categories of race and ethnicity.[14] Chang characterizes this divide as research that "privileges universal common risk factors, such as poverty, to explain group difference in mental illness versus . . . that which privileges group specific cultures, histories, and lived experience—such as racism [or colonialism] to explain group differences in mental illness" (Chang 2003, 379).[15] Despite these differences among researchers in minority mental health, culture counts continues to expand the relevance and develop new meanings of culture in psychiatry.

The Culture Counts movement was given further public exposure and its policy relevance enhanced by the publication of the Institute of Medicine's report, *Unequal Treatment: Confronting Racial and Ethnic Disparities in Healthcare* (2002–2003). The report presented a vast overview of National Institutes of Health (NIH) research from the decade of the 1990s that documented differences in treatment by race and ethnicity across a wide spectrum of medical and psychiatric conditions (Ayanian et al. 1999; Ayanian et al. 1993; Bach et al. 1999; Smedley, Stith, and Nelson 2003; Good et al. 2003; Waters 2008). For example, in psychiatry, differences were documented in diagnosis and medication practices, black men receiving misdiagnoses of greater severity more frequently than white men or women, and more frequently being prescribed older rather than newer psychopharmaceuticals.[16]

This genre of highly influential NIH research was nurtured by the successful political movements and ethnic-identity health-care politics of the late 1980s and early 1990s (Epstein 2007). In particular, the women's health movement and its congressional advocates, Patricia Schoeder and Olympia Snowe, successfully called for research on the diseases of women and minorities and explanations for differences by gender, race, and ethnicity in medical treatment for major disorders such as heart disease. In 1990, the force of law mandated inclusion of minorities and women in NIH-funded research (Kelty, Bates, and Pinn 2007, 130), bringing a virtual sea change in the research culture of NIH and along with it the findings of disparities in medical treatment.

Building on recent NIH research and motivated by its congressional charge, notably led by the Black Congressional Caucus, *Unequal Treatment* continued the critique of solely universalistic explanations for racial and ethnic differences in mental health care, providing evidence for a series of provocative and revolutionary arguments. It also demonstrated that differences in care for racial and ethnic minorities exist, even after taking into account universal, individual factors such as insurance status, access to care, and lifestyle choices. The authors referred to these remaining differences as disparities in care, which they tied to other more pernicious factors, such as clinician bias or racism. This dramatically shifted the terms of the debate away from the cultural characteristics of racial and ethnic minority members themselves to the culture and institutions of medicine itself—its individual clinicians and health-care providers, on medical education, training, research, and institutions of patient care—as sources of disparities in care.

Drawing from theories in social psychology on bias and stereotyping (Van Ryn 2002; Dovidio et al. 2008), *Unequal Treatment* emphasized personal bias and stereotyping within medicine as explanatory of disparities; yet it also implicated the broader culture of medicine and the medical gaze (Good et al. 2003; Good 1995a, 2001, 2007; Good and Hannah 2010; Good et al. 1990; Good et al. 1999). It recommended policies and interventions to redress clinician bias and to reduce disparities and inequalities in care by race and ethnicity. This shift in emphasis (and perhaps blame) from patient culture, race, and ethnicity to the culture of medicine found its way into twenty-first century NIH research agendas as well as into policies of health-care institutions and clinics. Centers for disparities research were soon established in many academic medical centers and teaching hospitals throughout the country, thereby following earlier developments of entrepreneurial adventures in cultural competence and diversity training that grew in response to the increasing cultural diversity of patient populations (Lo and Stacey 2008; Lakes, Lopez, and Garro 2006; Lopez 1997; Betancourt 2003, 2006; Guarnaccia and Rodriguez 1996; Kleinman and Benson 2006).

The cultural categories salient in these two national discussions— culture, race, and ethnicity for mental health, and race and ethnicity (and at times social class and gender) for disparities—have profoundly influenced the actions of health-care institutions and their clinicians and staff, shaping practices designed to respond to the increasing cultural hyperdiversity of patient populations and to reduce health-care and health disparities among disadvantaged ethnic and racial minorities. Culture counts and unequal treatment became the dominant policy themes defining in large measure the role culture plays in all its many meanings in medicine and psychiatry today.

However, the analytic categories of race and ethnicity underlying these dominant policy themes are being challenged by recent demographic trends that have brought increased immigration to the United States from around the world and exceptional residential mobility and racial and ethnic diversity in neighborhoods and cities and even rural communities across the country. Clinics once designed to serve primarily one ethnic community or a few neighborhood ethnic groups are now faced with a complex array of individuals from different and multiple ethnic backgrounds, speaking different languages, holding nuanced cultural perspectives, from different social classes, and with complicated historical experiences as well as racial and ethnic identities. These changes, which we refer to in this book as hyperdiversity, call for an expanded investigation of how culture counts in American mental health care. Culture may count in contemporary medicine and psychiatry, but in ways not well captured by the analytic research and policy categories that have relied solely on the mandated pentad of the national census. Cultural differences are vast among members of each of the major census categories, and each medical institution and profession has a unique cultural character and institutional history that powerfully shapes care in ways unrelated to simple definitions of race and ethnicity.

Curiously, the concept of culture as an analytic concept has increasingly been questioned by some anthropologists, just as health-care institutions and clinicians have increasingly routinized concepts and uses of culture as means for improving quality of care and reducing disparities, and as health-services researchers use culture as an independent variable to explain differences in health status and disparities in medical treatment. Anthropologists have grown concerned about the risks of essentializing societies (either as cultures plural, or subgroups within societies as subcultures) (Abu-Lughod 1991). A good deal of anthropological scholarship in recent years emphasizes how cultural communities and forms of cultural identity are variable, situational, dynamic, and embedded in struggles for power and control over resources. Our discussions of culture, both patients' culture and the culture of medicine, reflect the debates in anthropology (Goodale 2009; Marcus and Fischer 1999). Rather than throwing out the culture concept or judging it as outdated and of scant value, the chapters in this book caution against essentializing patient or ethnic group culture but acknowledge that culture, as well as ethnicity and race, continue to hold pragmatic significance for many people, and as such, requires continued attention from clinicians and social scientists.

Researching Psychiatry in Hyperdiverse Boston

Greater Boston, historically a major hub of immigration, continues to be a gateway city. Boston is historically unique as well in the distinctive boundary profiles of its ethnic communities and their links to the city's various health-care institutions—its community clinics, its hospitals, and its academic medical centers, which for decades had been publicly perceived as ethnically and religiously flavored. Strikingly, Boston's demographic transformation over the past three decades has dissolved many boundaries of ethnicity and religion that for generations characterized the culture and politics of Greater Boston and its segregated neighborhoods, ethnically defined (Bluestone and Stevenson 2000).[17] No longer predominantly Yankee, Brahman, Irish, Italian, African American, and Chinese; no longer just Catholic, Protestant, and Jewish; no longer black, white, and a little Asian; Boston's population of the twenty-first century has become a mosaic, a world city representing the diversity of the globe,[18] or what we refer to as a cultural environment of hyperdiversity.

Since 1970, Greater Boston has transformed from an environment in which blacks and whites made up 98 percent of the population to one in which whites are nearly the minority and Hispanics and Asians, combined, outnumber blacks. As figure 1.1 shows, the white population in Suffolk County[19] has declined from 84 percent in 1970 to just 52 percent in 2009 as immigration has rapidly increased and whites have continued their relocation to the suburbs (see also figure 1.2). As figure 1.3 shows, the foreign-born population in Suffolk County has doubled, from 13 percent in 1970 to nearly 26 percent in 2009. The black population in Suffolk County has grown moderately, increasing from 14 percent in 1970 to 20 percent in 2010, but its geographic distribution and ethnic composition has changed dramatically. Approximately half are now immigrants or children of immigrants from a growing number of countries in the Caribbean, Africa, and elsewhere[20] and, as figure 1.4 shows, now live in an expanding area south of the city from Roxbury through Dorchester, down to Mattapan, Roslindale, and Hyde Park. The Hispanic/Latino population has grown tremendously, increasing from just 3 percent in 1970 to 20 percent in 2010. A racially and ethnically diverse population of immigrants and refugees from throughout Latin America as well as American citizens originally from Puerto Rico, the Hispanic/Latino population is geographically widespread throughout Greater Boston and, as figure 1.5 shows, is particularly concentrated in cities and neighborhoods such as East Boston, Chelsea, and Jamaica Plain, where they are majorities or near majorities. The Asian population has also grown rapidly, increasing from less than 1 percent in 1970 to more than 8 percent in

Figure 1.1   Race-Ethnicity in Suffolk County, 1970 to 2010

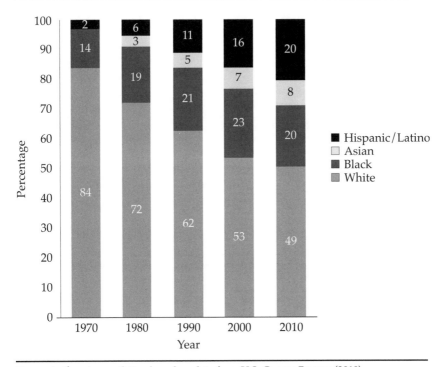

Source: Authors' compilation based on data from U.S. Census Bureau (2010).
Note: Data for Asian, black, and white exclude Hispanics/Latinos, who can be of any race.
Data also exclude individuals who marked more than one race.

2010, and as figure 1.6 shows, is no longer confined to Chinatown in central Boston. The Asian population has shifted in recent years to suburban areas, but significant ethnic enclaves exist; many Vietnamese live in Dorchester, and many Cambodians have settled in Lowell, outside Suffolk County.

As a result of these demographic shifts, the cultural identities of ethnic-specific clinics of past decades have changed radically, as have the ethnic and nativity profiles of both health-care staff and patient populations. Mission statements and ideologies of hospitals and medical centers have greater cultural flexibility, adapting to demographic changes by adding new culturally tailored services and languages as they appeal to an often rapidly changing demographic profile of new immigrant patients in their catchment areas while they continue to provide health-care services to more stable neighborhood populations (Hunter and Park 2010).

Figure 1.2   Percentage White in Suffolk County, 1970 to 2000

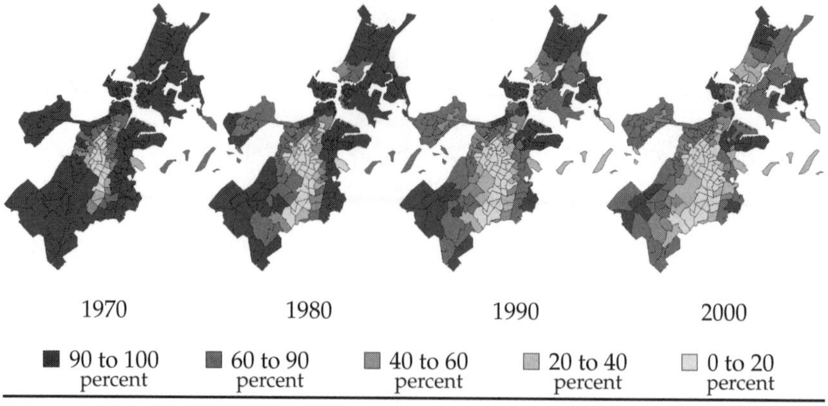

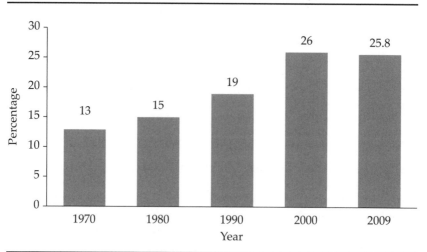

1970	1980	1990	2000

■ 90 to 100   ■ 60 to 90   ■ 40 to 60   □ 20 to 40   □ 0 to 20
percent   percent   percent   percent   percent

Source: Authors' compilation based on data from the U.S. Census Neighborhood Change Database (NCDB) 1970–2000 (GeoLytics 2010). Maps created with GeoLytics software.
Note: White population, with the exception of 1970, is non-Hispanic.

Figure 1.3   Percentage Foreign-Born in Suffolk County, 1970 to 2009

```
30

        26      25.8
25

                19
20

Percentage
        13      15
15

10

5

0
     1970   1980   1990   2000   2009
                   Year
```

Source: Authors' calculations based on data from the U.S. Census Bureau (2010).

Figure 1.4   Percentage Black in Suffolk County, 1970 to 2000

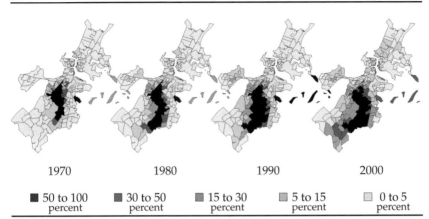

| 1970 | 1980 | 1990 | 2000 |

■ 50 to 100   ■ 30 to 50   ■ 15 to 30   ■ 5 to 15   ☐ 0 to 5
percent   percent   percent   percent   percent

Source: Authors' compilation based on data from the U.S. Census Neighborhood Change
Database (NCDB) 1970–2000 (GeoLytics 2010). Maps created with GeoLytics software.
Note: Black population, with the exception of 1970, is non-Hispanic.

Figure 1.5   Percentage Hispanic/Latino in Suffolk County, 1970 to 2000

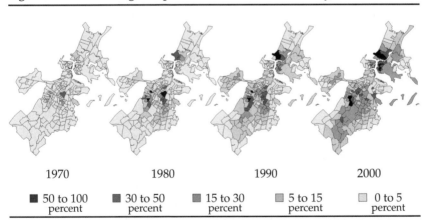

| 1970 | 1980 | 1990 | 2000 |

■ 50 to 100   ■ 30 to 50   ■ 15 to 30   ■ 5 to 15   ☐ 0 to 5
percent   percent   percent   percent   percent

Source: Authors' compilation based on data from the U.S. Census Neighborhood Change
Database (NCDB) 1970–2000 (GeoLytics 2010). Maps created with GeoLytics software.
Note: Hispanic population includes respondents of any race.

Figure 1.6   Percentage Asian in Suffolk County, 1980 to 2000

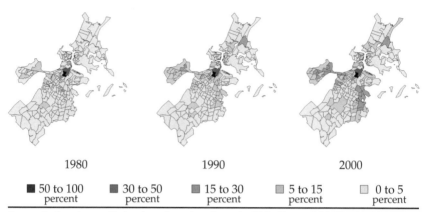

1980   1990   2000

■ 50 to 100   ■ 30 to 50   ■ 15 to 30   ▨ 5 to 15   ☐ 0 to 5
   percent   percent   percent   percent   percent

Source: Authors' compilation based on data from the U.S. Census Neighborhood Change Database (NCDB) 1970–2000 (GeoLytics 2010). Maps created with GeoLytics software.
Note: Asian population in 1980 is non-Hispanic/Latino, and includes American Indian, Asian, Native Hawaiian, and Pacific Islander. 1990 and 2000 do not include American Indian. Comparable data for 1970 were not available.

Many community clinics in Boston and neighboring towns are charged not only with providing care for established immigrant populations who have settled in their catchment area, but also with serving as a primary supportive institution for newly arrived refugees from a wide diversity of nations. Hub-and-spoke health-care systems, where the medical center is the hub and the community clinics are satellites (or feeders to the hub) dot Boston and its environs. These systems provide tertiary and high-technology medical care as well as ambulatory and primary care at the academic medical centers, plus primary care and outpatient services, including mental health services, at the community clinics. These organizational features pattern medical and psychiatric care throughout the Boston area and strongly influenced our research possibilities and site selections.

Greater Boston is also a major political player in the culture counts movement in mental health care and in the disparities movement to reduce inequalities in health status and treatment. In 2005, Mayor Thomas Menino charged the city's health-care institutions to redress disparities in health status and in healthcare following the publication of *Unequal Treatment*. As reported by Stephen Smith in the *Boston Globe* on June 23, 2005,

> Mayor Thomas M. Menino of Boston will unveil a comprehensive initiative this morning designed to address what public health authorities

regard as the city's most pressing medical issue: the intractable differences in health status between the races. As part of the 1 million dollar effort the city will help pay for hospitals to begin detailed tracking of racial and ethnic differences in the care patients receive, and it will underwrite training designed to make physicians more culturally sensitive. (B1)

Much of the research underpinning *Unequal Treatment* was produced by scholars from Boston's medical schools (Boston University, Harvard Medical School, Tufts Medical Center, and other institutions), and, building on their influence in national policy, centers for disparities research and cultural competence were established in Boston's academic medical centers (see Betancourt 2003, 2006; Ayanian et al. 1993; Ayanian et al. 1999; McGuire et al. 2006; Good et al. 2003). In addition, efforts to respond to the needs of new immigrant populations led Boston's clinical and hospital worlds to emphasize care designed to be culturally competent, sensitive, and appropriate.

Clinics, Clinicians, and Health-Care Staff

The anthropologists, sociologists, and psychiatrists who have written the chapters of *Shattering Culture* present innovative analyses of the work of culture and how it is invoked in the academic and community medical institutions and psychiatric clinics of Greater Boston. This interdisciplinary group of scholars conducted ethnographic observations and interviews with clinicians, health-care staff, and patients.

The research began with mapping current mental health services and clinical sites in Boston and environs, noting demographic and cultural transitions over the past three decades in each clinic's locales and patient populations, and transformations in clinical cultures, ownership, and governance.[21] We then created a typology of current clinics and psychiatric services: generic clinics and inpatient services, offering a range of interpreter and chaplain services, with universalistic identities and ideologies of care—the "we take everyone" sites; clinics with culturally specific identities and tailored services, such as the Latino clinic, staffed by Spanish-speaking clinicians and support staff; and community clinics identified by geographic neighborhood or place, offering a wide variety of language- and culturally specific care designed to serve highly diverse populations, including new immigrants. In phase one of the study, field methodologies were anthropological, including ethnographic observation and participant observation, as well as focused, open-ended interviews with clinicians and other health-care staff, and with patients and their physicians. Anthropological hanging out in a given research site often produces the best ethnographic field work, yet such methods are rarely tolerated in clinical settings. Thus, we chose clinical sites for our most intensive research where generous and frankly curious colleagues smoothed the way for this difficult field work.

We interviewed 192 health-care staff recruited from all ranks: psychiatrists, psychiatric residents, psychologists, social workers, nurses, front desk workers, clinic managers, interpreters, chaplains, patient advocates, and security guards. Our initial interview opened with a long question introducing core topics for our discussions, which usually lasted for an hour or longer. We interviewed some clinicians or staff more than once.

> [Introductory Script] We are interested in asking you some questions about the role of culture in the practice of medicine. We are trying to understand the experience of treating patients with various cultural backgrounds and practices, but we are also very interested in the culture of clinical practice itself: the way that your clinic is organized, how your day-to-day work is structured, the types of rules and procedures that are in place. We are interested in patient culture and what is sometimes referred to as organizational culture. Keep this in mind as we progress through the interview.

We analyzed interviews by deep reading and then, with the aid of data analysis software Atlas.ti©, we compared responses by site, profession, gender, and ethnicity. The clinical settings are described and presented in table 1.1; tables 1.2 through 1.4 present characteristics of interviewees. Across these clinical settings, we find a mosaic of difference by nativity, ethnicity, race, and language among clinicians and health-care staff, reflecting greater Boston's contemporary ethnic diversity.

Academic Medical Center Hub 1 (AMC1) is central to Boston's huge global reaching hub-and-spoke system. The academic medical center we refer to as AMC1 or the "mother ship" has cultural and interpreter services designed for both its global patients and for Greater Boston's patient populations. The granite walls of the main hospital lobby are engraved with uplifting statements about patient rights in twenty languages. AMC1's mission statement, revised in 2007 in response to Mayor Menino's charge, reads, "Guided by the needs of our patients and their families, we aim to deliver the very best health care . . . and to improve the health and well-being of the diverse communities we serve." We carried out observations and interviews with clinicians and staff at the hub in the acute psychiatric inpatient unit, in the psychiatric emergency department, and in the psychiatric outpatient department; we also interviewed interpreters and chaplains who served both psychiatric patients as well as other patients. Among the clinicians and staff interviewed, 75 percent self-identified as white, 9 percent as black, 5 percent as Asian American, 4 percent as multiracial, and 9 percent as Hispanic/Latino.

Table 1.1   Medical Sites and Psychiatric Clinics

Site	Clinic
Academic Medical Center 1 (AMC1)	Inpatient psychiatric unit Outpatient psychiatric service Acute psychiatric service (emergency department)
Academic Medical Center 2 (AMC2)	Outpatient Latino mental health clinic Psychiatric outpatient service Psychiatry residency training settings
Private Psychiatric Hospital (PPH)	Inpatient psychiatric unit
Neighborhood Community Health Center (NCHC)	Outpatient mental health services
Region Medical Center (RMC)	Outpatient and inpatient psychiatric services

Source: Authors' compilation.

Table 1.2   Phase 1: Number of Clinician and Staff Interviews by Site

All Sites	192
Academic Medical Center 1 (AMC1)	79
Academic Medical Center 2 (AMC2) and Latino Clinic	56
Neighborhood Community Health Center (NCHC)	24
Regional Medical Center (RMC)	19
Private Psychiatric Hospital (PPH)	14

Source: Authors' compilation.

The Neighborhood Community Clinic, a satellite of AMC1, has a long history of serving a highly diverse although constantly changing population of immigrants and minorities, and today its community is an environment characterized by ethnic and racial hyperdiversity. Its mental health clinic was established in 1978 in response to a fire that destroyed much of the small town. Its local outreach programs serve the poor and recent immigrants from many countries, including refugees fleeing political violence. Its patient population is very diverse, as is its mental health service staff. As a satellite community clinic, its staff complains at times—using a pejorative phrase commonly heard—that their clinic becomes the "dumping ground" for the AMC hub patients "with language needs" beyond the capacity of the hub clinicians. Linguistic capacity among clinicians includes Spanish, Somali, German, French, Portuguese, Italian, Serbo-Croatian,

Table 1.3   Number of Interviews by Profession

Total interviews	192
Psychiatrists, psychologists, and other M.D.s M.D. psychiatrists, Ph.D. psychologists, other M.D.s, other Ph.D.s	74
Other mental health professionals Social workers, mental health counselors with master's degree	27
Other health-care staff Nurses, mental health workers, occupational therapists, dieticians	27
Patient support staff Interpreters, chaplains, advocates, mental health associates	47
Administrative support staff Security, housekeeping, dietary, clerical	11
Management support staff Nonmedical administrative and clerical managers	6

Source: Authors' compilation.

Table 1.4   Phase 1: Clinician and Staff Interview Demographics (N=192)

Gender	Female	66%
	Male	34%
Age	Mean years (SD)	Range
	43.16 (12.3)	21–70
Origin	White	68%
	Black, African American	12%
	Asian	7%
	Multiracial	3%
	Other	10%
Ethnicity	Hispanic, Latino	14%
	Not Hispanic, Latino	86%
Foreign-born or Puerto Rican–born		29%
U.S.-born		71%

Source: Authors' compilation.

Afrikaans, Hindi, and Gujarati. Medical interpreters for other languages are also accessible. This language and cultural capacity helps create an environment to which patients are willing to return. We interviewed mental health clinicians and staff from the mental health clinic as well as interpreters serving all medical and mental health units. Sixty-three percent of clinicians and staff interviewed self-identified as white,

14 percent as black, 5 percent as Asian, 18 percent as other, and 27 percent as ethnically Hispanic.

Academic Medical Center 2 (AMC2) is a collection of teaching hospitals and academic medical programs. The mergers of hospitals have wrought havoc with previously strong and distinctive cultural identities and ideologies of clinical practice and nursing care (Weinberg 2003). The Latino clinic is an outpatient psychiatric clinic specifically designed to care for Spanish-speaking patients with Spanish-speaking clinicians and support staff; however, because the hospital offers excellent primary care and draws patients from the Greater Boston area, the Latino clinic is not a bounded site, and clinicians from the Latino team also care for patients who do not identify themselves as Latino or Hispanic. The clinic mission was established by its director, a psychiatrist who also trains residents and educates clinicians in culture and psychiatry and cultural competence. Clinicians, staff, and trainees were interviewed, as were patients. Twelve percent of clinicians and staff interviewed self-identified their race as black, 3 percent as Asian, 12 percent as multiracial, and 73 percent as white; 24 percent self-identified their ethnicity as Hispanic/Latino.

The Private Psychiatric Hospital (PPH) is unique; it takes all patients and is professionally known as the mental hospital of last resort for Boston area patients for whom beds are unavailable at other institutions. It serves many patients who are poor. Nonetheless, its Joint Commission rating rivals those of the academic medical centers' hub hospitals. Its patient population is ethnically and racially diverse, and some units are labeled with cultural designations, such as a Hispanic group, but the categorization often does not coincide with patient self-identification. Clinicians and staff interviewed self-identified as 36 percent white, 50 percent black (half of whom were immigrants from Africa), and 14 percent as Asian or Asian Americans.

The Regional Medical Center is part of the hub-and-spoke system in which the regional center is a larger satellite. The hospital's mental health services include inpatient and outpatient clinics with a local reach. Although suburban, it serves poor as well as middle-class patients, including recent immigrants. Clinicians and staff we interviewed practiced in both inpatient and outpatient psychiatric services. Eighty-eight percent of those interviewed self-identified as white, 12 percent as other; 10 percent of those self-identifying as white identified as ethnically Hispanic.

Interviews with Psychiatric Patients

In phase two of the study, fifty patients and selected providers from inpatient or outpatient psychiatric clinical settings were interviewed; others also participated in discussions with ethnographers. Patients were asked about their illness and care, and about how culture mattered in their treatment. Most patients interviewed were highly experienced with psychiatric cultures and openly discussed the benefits, gains, and negative and positive experiences with their various clinics and their clinicians. Interviews ranged between twenty minutes to over an hour and were transcribed and analyzed, also with the aid of Atlas.ti. The patient population, like the provider population, is racially and ethnically diverse, reflecting greater Boston's current demographics. Thirty percent were born outside the United States, 65 percent self-identified racially as white, 9 percent as black, 26 percent as other; 26 percent of the total self-identified as Hispanic or Latino; ages ranged from eighteen to eighty-four. Thirty percent were covered by private insurance, and 66 percent by Mass Health, Commonwealth Care, or Medicare.

The Book

The chapters draw both on author interviews and observations, and narrative analyses of case studies, as well as from the study's larger data set and qualitative analyses of multiple interviews. Each chapter explores themes and questions central to the project's overall investigation and research design, and interprets findings which emerged out of analyses of the empirical data, the interviews and observations, and the ethnographic hanging out.

Cultural Environments of Hyperdiversity

Part I paints a complex portrait of culture and its manifold meanings, roles, and implications in medical as well as psychiatric clinical settings of Greater Boston. In chapter 2, Seth Hannah, a sociologist specializing in social inequality and cultural studies of medicine, sets the stage for our discussion, introducing the book's motivating concepts of hyperdiversity and cultural environments of hyperdiversity. These terms convey two core meanings. First, hyperdiversity offers a way of describing the increasingly diverse nature of patient populations in contemporary American healthcare settings. Given the heterogeneity within social groups, patient populations cannot be grouped or classified only according to superficial features like phenotype, mother tongue, or nationality. In its second sense, cultural environments of hyperdiversity describes particular social settings in which complex interactions among multiple forms of difference and diversity—for instance, race, ethnicity, culture, gender, sexual orientation, and socioeconomic class—intersect in ways that significantly influence efforts to cultivate clinical rapport and trust. The term *hyperdiversity* captures those situations in which the link between racial-ethnic identity and culture is weak or broken (shattered) and, as a result, in which broad, identity-based indicators of cultural difference prove too blunt an instrument for navigating the social heterogeneity within today's clinical environments.

The three subsequent chapters explore three strategies employed within American health care settings in response to these cultural environments of hyperdiversity: interpreter services, chaplain services, and clinician-patient matching. In chapter 3, Sarah Willen, an anthropologist of immigration and medical anthropology, explores the apparent dilemma that an increased commitment by health-care institutions to provide interpreter services, often supported by state mandates and institutional funding, does not necessarily resolve the clinical challenges associated with language barriers, often because clinicians have limited familiarity or experience discomfort with their institutions' prevailing models of clinical interpretation. Chapter 3 characterizes the largely unchoreographed dance among patient, interpreter, and clinician, the often ambiguous role of interpreters, and their frustrations with clinicians who just don't get it. In chapter 4, Lisa Stevenson, a cultural anthropologist specializing in medical anthropology, explores how chaplaincy comes to be seen as a cultural service in major medical centers, noting that "to know how culture counts we need to know what counts as culture." Stevenson explains how the potential divisiveness of religious difference has largely been reworked into a cultural difference both palatable and comprehensible to hospital bureaucracies. Despite the challenging translational work that leaves many chaplains "praying along"—at times uncomfortably—with people who do not share their faith, their services are nonetheless consistently identified by other hospital staff as an institutional attempt to provide culturally sensitive care. A third strategy, which Willen considers in chapter 5, addresses the technique of matching patients with providers who share their cultural or racial-ethnic backgrounds. Although clinician-patient matching was touted in the 1990s, especially in mental health, the clinicians we interviewed are generally unconvinced of its singular value for either improving clinician-patient rapport or remediating disparities in mental health outcomes.

Clinical Cultures, Clinical Realities

Part II takes us into the dizzying worlds of psychiatry and mental health practice in Greater Boston. Drawing on interviews with psychiatrists, other mental health clinicians and support staff, and patients, as well as on author experiences as psychiatrists, these chapters feature a unique mix of insider and outsider perspectives on contemporary clinical realities in cultural environments of hyperdiversity. Chapter 6, by Sarah S. Willen, Seth Hannah, Ken Vickery, and Mary-Jo DelVecchio Good, with psychiatrist-researcher Marina Yaroshenko, traces the personal journey of Dr. Z. through emigration from the former Soviet Union to a professional journey through multiple American training residencies, each stressing different therapeutic models from psychodynamic to biological modalities of diagnosis and therapeutics. In chapter 7, Sadeq Rahimi, a scholar of cultural psychiatry, Seth Hannah, and Mary-Jo DelVecchio Good illustrate how the practice of modern psychiatry is not a closed culture but is instead shaped by a number of external factors in the social, political, and institutional environment. Using the notion of cultural traffic, they find that global flows of knowledge—the growing cosmopolitan and biomedical nature of modern psychiatry—and global flows of people—increasing hyperdiversity among patient populations and practicing psychiatrists—combine to shape local forms of clinical practice.

Cultural and interpersonal dynamics and how they influence the perspectives and experiences of patients are addressed in chapters 8 and 9. In chapter 8, Elizabeth Carpenter-Song, a psychological anthropologist who specializes in the lived experiences of patients in psychiatric treatment, as well as those of their families, engages with American psychiatry as a moral enterprise, attending to the on-the-ground realities of clinicians and patients, and asks what one is to make of happy patients. Carpenter-Song argues that we have much to learn from patients' positive experiences, and that recognition—the "who are you" question—is crucial to positive therapeutic relationships in mental health care, regardless of patient ethnicity and diversity or patient-provider matching. In chapter 9, Joseph Calabrese, anthropologist and psychotherapist, explores the flip side of this question, the negative as well as positive experiences in two psychiatric in-patient services, one in Boston and one in the Midwest. Calabrese also finds that recognition of the patient as a person and the quality of clinician interaction is of ultimate importance, and that a single dismissive interaction can lead patients to distrust an entire institution or even an entire professional discipline. He also notes that patients spoke about experiencing discrimination from physicians other than psychiatrists—not on the basis of race or gender but instead of the stigma of mental illness.

The book's final chapters offer a sobering window into the real-life, day-to-day culture of psychiatry by revealing how challenges posed by cultural environments of hyperdiversity are often eclipsed by growing administrative, bureaucratic, and economic demands and constraints. Here, we as researchers and authors ask, "Does economy trump culture?" In chapter 10, cultural psychiatrist Antonio Bullon collaborates with Good and Carpenter-Song to analyze how paperwork and documentation—cultures of practice driven by the technological mode so salient today in medicine—have become increasingly regarded by clinicians as burdens imposed by outside forces intruding on clinic time and therapeutic work with patients. This burden is especially true for psychiatrists treating disadvantaged and minority patients, who are most likely to require not just care for mental health and medical problems, but also assistance in meeting social needs. The technical rationality driving documentation practices emerges in even starker relief in chapter 11, by Hannah and Good, in collaboration with the psychiatrist and anthropologist Lawrence T. Park. The authors highlight the anxiety and frustrations that psychiatrists, mental health clinicians, clinic directors, and patients experience when confronted with a maze of insurance and financial regulations both public and private. Clinicians in our study speak about their frustrations especially when their patients get stuck because of financial constraints.

This last chapter foregrounds one of the book's central insights. Although hyperdiversity poses substantial challenges to psychiatry and the entire medical commons, we find that individuals and institutions readily rise to redress problems of disparities and to enhance culturally competent or sensitive and quality care for Greater Boston's mosaic of patient populations. The authors find, however, that economic complexity complicates these efforts, at times posing far greater challenges to providing equitable mental health care for minorities and disadvantaged patients than any due to cultural difference.

Notes

1. Many institutions of academic medicine, community health clinics, and nonprofit medical centers and charity and religious hospitals, and even for-profit hospitals seeking Medicaid and Medicare and other public funding, required attention to cultural distinctions, in particular the requirement that patients had a right to interpreter services. This can also be seen as a marketing issue to reach out to the widest possible patient population.
2. 1970, 1980, 1990, 2000, and 2010 Censuses (U.S. Census Bureau, various years).
3. These questions resonate with the foundation's program in culture contact and more specifically in immigration and ethnicity. The many publications on immigration and culture contact from the RSF series and research programs are relevant here (see, for example, Waters 1999; Kasinitz et al. 2008; Bluestone and Stevenson 2000; Shweder, Minow, and Markus 2004; Hochschild 1995; Hochschild and Powell 2008; Suárez-Orozco and Páez 2003; Bean and Stevens 2003).
4. These were part of the OEO projects of President Johnson's Great Society movement.
5. The Race Remixed series in the *New York Times* focuses on how the growing population that self-identifies as multiracial is blurring contemporary notions of race and ethnicity in America (see Susan Saulny, "Black? White? Asian? More Young Americans Choose All of the Above," *New York Times,* January 29, 2011).
6. Susan Saulny's *New York Times* article, "Multiracial Nation, Many Ways to Tally" (2011) is an example of hyperdiversity. Uncertainty about an individual's culture, race, and ethnicity is common among many young Americans

who check all or other. Ms. M., who is part Irish, Peruvian, Chinese, Cherokee and Shawnee, is categorized differently depending on who is counting. Her father calls her Hispanic, she and her mother prefer to use other, and her best friend uses mixed race; in the census she can use four races, with the U.S. Department of Education she would be Hispanic, and with the National Center for Health Statistics she would be Asian.

7. UC Davis had a cultural consultation clinic of which we (Mary-Jo and Byron Good) were a part.

8. Many conversations with members of the DSM V working group on culture included psychiatrists Roberto Lewis-Fernandez, Devon Hinton, and Anne Becker (March 2009, November 2009, January 2010, and March 2011).

9. The DSM III Case Book (Spitzer et al. 1981) included eighty-seven cases that were 75 percent white professionals, wealthy business people, or members of the middle class; 15 percent prisoners or unemployed or elderly; and 11 percent working class; one case suggested a Hispanic ethnic identity (Good 1993). In the DSM IV, 20 percent of male adults were marked by a race or ethnicity, while 13 percent of women were (Spitzer 1994; Cermele, Daniels, and Anderson 2001).

10. This is a paraphrase of a comment by Michael Jackson on understanding the human condition and learning how to live with others as an anthropologist. William James Hall, Harvard University, April 15, 2011.

11. A cultural change in psychiatry from roman numerals to Arabic and digital formats allows for possible changes without changing the identifying numeral—that is, 5.0, 5.1 and so on.

12. By the mid-twentieth century, as massive mental hospitals and asylums began to be regarded as inhumane and deinstitutionalization became the norm, the community health movement began to flourish. Although many mentally ill patients had legitimate reasons to fear and distrust the asylum psychiatry of the mid-twentieth century and the stigmata taint of hospitalization, with the establishment of community mental health services and a sea change in medication options, the treatment for mental illness was less onerous.

13. Joe Gone's October 2011 conference at the University of Michigan has culture counts as its theme. The conference, titled *Reconciling Cultural Competence & Evidence-Based Practice in Mental Health Services,* featured contributions by leading experts in the field of culture and psychiatry (psychiatrists, anthropologists, and health services researchers). Culture and psychiatry go together, and the meaning of each has been dynamic and fluid. For many years, the National Institute of Mental Health actively supported basic research and training programs, including those for anthropologists in culture and psychiatry. Harvard's training program in Culture and Mental Health Services Research (MH 18006), directed for twenty-four years by Byron Good, Arthur Kleinman, and Mary-Jo Good, supported the postdoctoral fellows who contributed to the project described in this book.

The classic literature in anthropology, culture, and psychiatry is far too vast to be fully referenced here. Several notable publications include Mezzich et al.'s *Culture & Psychiatric Diagnosis: A DSM-IV Perspective* (1996), anthropologically important studies, including Kleinman and Good's *Culture and*

Depression (1986), Kleinman's *Rethinking Psychiatry* (1991), and Luhrmann's *Of Two Minds* (2000). Ethnographic classics include Estroff's *Making It Crazy* (1981), Rhodes's *Emptying Beds* (1995), and the sociological classic *Asylums* by Goffman (1961). More recent ethnographic work appears in collections such as Jenkins and Barrett's *Schizophrenia, Culture, and Subjectivity* (2004), Hinton and Good's *Culture and Panic Disorder* (2009), and Jenkins's *The Pharmaceutical Self* (2011). *Culture, Medicine and Psychiatry,* a journal of cross-cultural and comparative research (founded by Arthur Kleinman in 1977), was edited by Byron and Mary-Jo Good from 1986 through 2004, with Anne Becker, Peter Guarnaccia, and Roberto Lewis-Fernandez through 2006, and currently by Atwood Gaines since 2007. It has been a central academic journal in this field.

Despite this interest in culture, psychiatry has also had significant blind spots and disparities and inequalities in treatment by race, especially black and white, are documented in IOM's *Unequal Treatment,* in Good et al.'s *Unequal Treatment* (2003), and in Jonathan Metzl's *The Protest Psychosis* (2009).

14. A tension between universalism and cultural particularism is a different form of dualism, yet recalls Tanya Luhrmann's cultural analysis of psychiatry's duality between bioscience and biologically grounded psychiatric practice and psychodynamic therapeutics and practice, in her ethnography, *Of Two Minds* (2000).

15. See 2003 special issue of *Culture, Medicine and Psychiatry* (CMP), *The Politics of Science: Culture, Race, Ethnicity* and the *Supplement to the Surgeon General's Report on Mental Health,* edited by Doris Chang, Mary-Jo Good, and Byron Good; authors of essays in CMP tell the story of their contributions to the Surgeon General's supplement, *Mental Health: Culture, Race and Ethnicity* (Chang, Good, and Good 2003; Lopez 2003; Manson 2003; Miranda, Nakamura, and Bernal 2003; Richardson, Flaherty, and Bell 2003; Satcher 2003; Snowden 2003; Sue and Chu 2003; Takeuchi and Gage 2003).

16. There is some debate over which drugs are best, but African American men were less likely to be prescribed the most recent innovative psychopharmaceuticals (Good et al. 2003).

17. William Foote Whyte, Street Corner Society, 1954.

18. Workshop comment, April 29, 2009.

19. Suffolk County is comprised of the city of Boston and its surrounding communities, and is a good proxy for Greater Boston.

20. Between 2000 and 2006, the number of residents in the city of Boston from Haiti increased 6 percent, from Jamaica 13 percent, and from various African countries 52 percent.

21. Ownership shifted from community to academic medical centers for some Community Health Clinics; clinics were also absorbed into the Partners and CareGroup complexes.

References

Abu-Lughod, Lila. 1991. "Writing Against Culture." In *Recapturing Anthropology: Working in the Present,* edited by Richard G. Fox. Santa Fe, N.M.: School of American Research Press.

Anderson, Warwick, Deborah Jenson, and Richard C. Keller, eds. 2011. *Unconscious Dominions: Psychoanalysis, Colonial Trauma, and Global Sovereignties.* Durham, N.C.: Duke University Press.

Ayanian, John Z., Paul D. Cleary, Joel S. Weissman, and Arnold M. Epstein. 1999. "The Effect of Patients' Preferences on Racial Differences in Access to Renal Transplantation." *New England Journal of Medicine* 341(22): 1661–669.

Ayanian, John Z., I. Steven Udvarhelyi, Constantine A. Gatsonis, Chris L. Pasho, and Arnold M. Epstein. 1993. "Racial Differences in the Use of Revascularization Procedures after Coronary Angiography." *Journal of the American Medical Association* 269(20): 2642–646.

Bach, Peter B., Laura F. D. Cramer, Joan L. Warren, and Colin B. Begg. 1999. "Racial Differences in the Treatment of Early-Stage Lung Cancer." *New England Journal of Medicine* 341(16): 1198–205.

Bean, Frank D., and Gillian Stevens. 2003. *America's Newcomers and the Dynamics of Diversity.* New York: Russell Sage Foundation.

Betancourt, Joseph R. 2003. "Cross-Cultural Medical Education: Conceptual Approaches and Frameworks for Evaluation." *Academic Medicine* 78(6): 560–69.

———. 2006. "Cultural Competence and Medical Education: Many Names, Many Perspectives, One Goal." *Academic Medicine* 81(6): 499–501.

Bluestone, Barry, and Mary Huff Stevenson. 2000. *The Boston Renaissance: Race, Space, and Economic Change in an American Metropolis.* New York: Russell Sage Foundation.

Centers for Disease Control and Prevention (CDC). 2011. "Health Disparities and Inequalities Report, United States." *Morbidity and Mortality Weekly Report:* January 14.

Cermele, Jill A., Sharon Daniels, and Kristin L. Anderson. 2001. "Defining Normal: Constructions of Race and Gender in the DSM-IV Casebook." *Feminism & Psychology* 11(2): 229–47.

Chang, Doris F. 2003. "An Introduction to the Politics of Science: Culture, Race, Ethnicity and the Supplement to the Surgeon General's Report on Mental Health." *Culture, Medicine and Psychiatry* 27(4): 373–83.

Chang, Doris F., Mary-Jo DelVecchio Good, and Byron J. Good. 2003. "The Politics of Science: Culture, Race, Ethnicity, and the Supplement to the Surgeon General's Report on Mental Health." Special issue, *Culture, Medicine and Psychiatry* 27(4).

Dovidio, John F., Louis A. Penner, Terrance L. Albrecht, Wynne E. Norton, Samuel L. Gartner, and J. Nicole Shelton. 2008. "Disparities and Distrust." *Social Science & Medicine* 67(3): 478–86.

Epstein, Steven. 2007. *Inclusion: The Politics of Difference in Medical Research.* Chicago: University of Chicago Press.

Estroff, Sue. 1981. *Making It Crazy.* Berkeley: University of California Press.

Geolytics. 2010. *Census CD Neighborhood Change Database [NCDB] Tract Data from 1970–2000.* East Brunswick, N.J.: Geolytics, Inc.

Goffman, Erving. 1961. *Asylums.* Garden City, N.Y.: Anchor Books.

Good, Byron J. 1993. "Culture, Diagnosis, and Comorbidity." *Culture, Medicine and Psychiatry* 16(4): 427–46.

Good, Byron J., and Mary-Jo DelVecchio Good. 1980. "The Meaning of Symptoms: A Cultural Hermeneutic Model for Clinical Practice." In *The Relevance of Social Science for Medicine.* Dordrecht, Neth.: D. Reidel.

———. 2010. "Amok in Java: Madness and Violence in Indonesian Politics." In *A Reader in Medical Anthropology: Theoretical Trajectories, Emergent Realities,* edited by Byron J. Good, Michael Fischer, Sarah Willen, and Mary-Jo DelVecchio Good. Hoboken, N.J.: Wiley-Blackwell.

Good, Mary-Jo DelVecchio. 1995a. *American Medicine: The Quest for Competence.* Berkeley: University of California Press.

———. 1995b. "Cultural Studies of Biomedicine: An Agenda for Research." *Social Science & Medicine* 41(4): 461–73.

———. 2001. "The Biotechnical Embrace." *Culture, Medicine and Psychiatry* 25(4): 395–410.

———. 2007. "The Medical Imaginary and the Biotechnical Embrace." In *Subjectivity,* edited by João Guilherme Biehl, Byron Good, and Arthur Kleinman. Berkeley: University of California Press.

Good, Mary-Jo DelVecchio, Byron J. Good, Cynthia Schaffer, and Stuart E. Lind. 1990. "American Oncology and the Discourse on Hope." *Culture, Medicine, and Psychiatry* 14(1): 59–79.

Good, Mary-Jo DelVecchio, Cara James, Byron J. Good, and Anne E. Becker. 2003. "The Culture of Medicine and Racial, Ethnic, and Class Disparities in Healthcare." In *Unequal Treatment: Confronting Racial and Ethnic Disparities in Health Care,* edited by Brian D. Smedley, Adrienne Y. Stith, and Alan R. Nelson. Washington, D.C.: National Academies Press.

Good, Mary-Jo DelVecchio, and Seth Hannah. 2010. "Medical Cultures." In *Handbook of Cultural Sociology,* edited by John R. Hall, Laura Grindstaff, and Ming-Cheng M. Lo. London: Routledge.

Good, Mary-Jo DelVecchio, Esther Mwaikambo, Erastus Amayo, and James M'Imunya Machoki. 1999. "Clinical Realities and Moral Dilemmas: Contrasting Perspectives from Academic Medicine in Kenya, Tanzania, and America." *Daedalus* 128(4): 167–96.

Goodale, Mark. 2009. *Surrendering to Utopia: An Anthropology of Human Rights.* Palo Alto, Calif.: Stanford University Press.

Guarnaccia, Peter, and Orlando Rodriguez. 1996. "'Concepts of Culture and Their Role in the Development of Culturally-Competent Mental Health Services." *Hispanic Journal of Behavioral Sciences* 18(4): 419–43.

Hannah, Seth. 2011. "Clinical Care in Environments of Hyper-Diversity: Race, Culture, and Ethnicity in the Post-Pentad World." Ph.D. dissertation. Department of Sociology, Harvard University.

Hinton, Devon, and Byron J. Good. 2009. *Culture and Panic Disorder.* Palo Alto, Calif.: Stanford University Press.

Hochschild, Jennifer L. 1995. *Facing Up to the American Dream: Race, Class, and the Soul of the Nation.* Princeton, N.J.: Princeton University Press.

Hochschild, Jennifer L., and Brenna M. Powell. 2008. "Racial Reorganization and the United States Census 1850–1930: Mulattoes, Half-Breeds, Mixed Parentage, Hindoos, and the Mexican Race." *Studies in American Political Development* 22(1): 59–96.

Hunter, Mary-Lyons, and Lawrence T. Park. 2010. "Gateway Communities: Providing Healthcare, Negotiating Citizenship for New Immigrant Populations." Unpublished manuscript.

Jenkins, Janis H., ed. 2011. *Pharmaceutical Self: The Global Shaping of Experience in an Age of Psychopharmacology.* Santa Fe, N.M.: School for Advanced Research Press.

Jenkins, Janis H., and Robert Barrett. 2004. *Schizophrenia, Culture, and Subjectivity: The Edge of Experience.* Cambridge: Cambridge University Press.

Kasinitz, Philip, John Mollenkopf, Mary C. Waters, and Jennifer Holdway. 2008. *Inheriting the City: The Children of Immigrants Come of Age.* New York: Russell Sage Foundation / Cambridge, Mass.: Harvard University Press.

Kelty, Miriam, Angela Bates, and Vivian W. Pinn. 2007. "National Institutes of Health Policy on the Inclusion of Women and Minorities as Subjects in Clinical Research." In *Principles and Practice of Clinical Research,* edited by John Gallin and Frederick P. Ognibene. Boston, Mass.: Elsevier/Academic Press.

Kleinman, Arthur. 1991. *Rethinking Psychiatry.* New York: The Free Press.

Kleinman, Arthur, and Peter Benson. 2006. "Anthropology in the Clinic: The Problem of Cultural Competency and How to Fix It." *PLos Medicine* 3(10): 1673–76.

Kleinman, Arthur, and Byron J. Good. 1986. *Culture and Depression.* Berkeley: University of California Press.

Kleinman, Arthur, Leon Eisenberg, and Byron J. Good. 1978. "Culture, Illness, and Care: Clinical Lessons from Anthropologic and Cross-Cultural Research." *Annals of Internal Medicine* 88(2): 251–58.

Lakes, Kimberly, Steven Lopez, and Linda C. Garro. 2006. "Cultural Competence and Psychotherapy: Applying Anthropologically Informed Conceptions of Culture." *Psychotherapy: Theory Research, Practice, Training* 43(4): 380–96.

Lee, Jennifer, and Frank D. Bean. 2010. *The Diversity Paradox: Immigration and the Color Line in the 21st Century.* New York: Russell Sage Foundation Press.

Lo, Ming-Cheng M., and Clare L. Stacey. 2008. "Beyond Cultural Competency: Bourdieu, Patients and Clinical Encounters." *Sociology of Health & Illness* 30(5): 741–55.

Lopez, Steven R. 1997. "Cultural Competence in Psychotherapy: A Guide for Clinicians and Their Supervisors." In *Handbook of Psychotherapy Supervision,* edited by C. Edward Watkins Jr. Hoboken, N.J.: John Wiley & Sons.

———. 2003. "Reflections on the Surgeon General's Report on Mental Health, Culture, Race, and Ethnicity." In "The Politics of Science: Culture, Race, Ethnicity, and the Supplement to the Surgeon General's Report on Mental Health," edited by Doris F. Chang, Mary-Jo DelVecchio Good, and Byron J. Good. Special issue, *Culture, Medicine and Psychiatry* 27(4): 419–34.

Luhrmann, Tanya M. 2000. *Of Two Minds.* New York: Alfred A. Knopf.

Manson, Spero M. 2003. "Extending the Boundaries, Bridging the Gaps: Crafting Mental Health: Culture, Race, and Ethnicity, a Supplement to the Surgeon General's Report on Mental Health." In "The Politics of Science: Culture, Race, Ethnicity, and the Supplement to the Surgeon General's Report on Mental Health," edited by Doris F. Chang, Mary-Jo DelVecchio Good, and Byron J. Good. Special issue, *Culture, Medicine, and Psychiatry* 27(4): 395–408.

Marcus, George E., and Michael M. J. Fischer. 1999. *Anthropology as Cultural Critique: An Experimental Moment in the Human Sciences.* Chicago: University of Chicago Press.

McGuire, Thomas G., Margarita Alegria, Benjamin L. Cook, Kenneth B. Wells, and Alan M. Zaslavsky. 2006. "Implementing the Institute of Medicine Definition of Disparities: An Application to Mental Health Care." *Health Services Research* 41(5): 1979–2005.

Metzl, Jonathan M. 2009. *The Protest Psychosis: How Schizophrenia Became a Black Disease.* Boston: Beacon Press.

Mezzich, Juan, Arthur Kleinman, Horacio Fabrega, and Delores Parron. 1996. *Culture & Psychiatric Diagnosis: A DSM-IV Perspective.* Washington, D.C.: American Psychiatric Press.

Miranda, Jeanne, Richard Nakamura, and Guillermo Bernal. 2003. "Including Ethnic Minorities in Mental Health Intervention Research: A Practical Approach to a Long Standing Problem." In "The Politics of Science: Culture, Race, Ethnicity, and the Supplement to the Surgeon General's Report on Mental Health," edited by Doris F. Chang, Mary-Jo DelVecchio Good, and Byron J. Good. Special issue, *Culture, Medicine and Psychiatry* 27(4): 467–86.

Pols, Hans. 2011. "The Totem Vanishes, the Hordes Revolt: A Psychoanalytic Interpretation of the Indonesian Struggle for Independence." In *Unconscious Dominions: Psychoanalysis, Colonial Trauma, and Global Sovereignties,* edited by Warwick Anderson, Deborah Jenson, and Richard C. Keller. Durham, N.C.: Duke University Press.

Prewitt, Kenneth. 2005. "Racial Classification in America: Where Do We Go from Here?" *Daedalus* 134(1): 5–17.

———. 2009. "Does (Should) Racial Counting Have a Future in America?" Lecture presented at the John F. Kennedy School of Government, Harvard University. Cambridge, Mass. (February 23).

Rhodes, Lorna. 1995. *Emptying Beds.* Berkeley and Los Angeles: University of California Press.

Richardson, Jerome, Tanya Anderson, Joseph Flaherty, and Carl Bell. 2003. "The Quality of Mental Health Care for African Americans." In "The Politics of Science: Culture, Race, Ethnicity, and the Supplement to the Surgeon General's Report on Mental Health," edited by Doris F. Chang, Mary-Jo DelVecchio Good, and Byron J. Good. Special issue, *Culture, Medicine and Psychiatry* 27(4): 487–98.

Satcher, David. 2001. "Commentary: Message from the 16th Surgeon General." In "The Politics of Science: Culture, Race, Ethnicity, and the Supplement to the Surgeon General's Report on Mental Health," edited by Doris F. Chang, Mary-Jo DelVecchio Good, and Byron J. Good. Special issue, *Culture, Medicine and Psychiatry* 27(4): 385–86.

Saulny, Susan. 2011. "Multiracial Nation, Many Ways to Tally." *New York Times,* February 10, 2011.

Shweder, Richard A., Martha Minow, and Hazel Rose Markus, eds. 2004. *Engaging Cultural Differences: The Multicultural Challenge in Liberal Democracies.* New York: Russell Sage Foundation.

Smedley, Brian D., Adrienne Y. Stith, and Alan Ray Nelson, eds. 2003. *Unequal Treatment: Confronting Racial and Ethnic Disparities in Health Care.* Washington, D.C.: National Academies Press.

Snowden, Lonnie R. 2003. "Challenges to Consensus in Preparing the Supplement to the Surgeon General's Report on Mental Health." In "The Politics of Science: Culture, Race, Ethnicity, and the Supplement to the Surgeon General's Report on Mental Health," edited by Doris F. Chang, Mary-Jo DelVecchio Good, and Byron J. Good. Special issue, *Culture, Medicine and Psychiatry* 27(4): 409–18.

Spitzer, Robert L., Andrew E. Skodol, Miriam Gibbon, and Janet B. W. Williams. 1981. *DSM-III Casebook*. Washington, D.C.: American Psychiatric Association.

Spitzer, Robert L., Miriam Gibbon, Andrew E. Skodol, Janet B. W. Williams, and Michael B. First, eds. 1994. *DSM-IV Casebook*. Washington, D.C.: American Psychiatric Press.

Suárez-Orozco, Marcelo M., and Mariela Páez, eds. 2003. *Latinos: Remaking America*. Cambridge, Mass.: David Rockefeller Center for Latin American Studies at Harvard University / Berkeley: University of California Press.

Suárez-Orozco, Marcelo M., Carola Suárez-Orozco, and Desirée Baolian Qin, eds. 2005. *The New Immigration: An Interdisciplinary Reader*. New York: Routledge.

Sue, Stanley. 1977. "Community Mental Health Services to Minority Groups: Some Optimism, Some Pessimism." *American Psychologist* 32(8): 616–24.

———. 1998. "In Search of Cultural Competence in Psychotherapy and Counseling." *American Psychologist* 53(4): 440–48.

Sue, Stanley, and June Y. Chu. 2003. "The Mental Health of Ethnic Minority Groups: Challenges Posed by the Supplement to the Surgeon General's Report on Mental Health." In "The Politics of Science: Culture, Race, Ethnicity, and the Supplement to the Surgeon General's Report on Mental Health," edited by Doris F. Chang, Mary-Jo DelVecchio Good, and Byron J. Good. Special issue, *Culture, Medicine and Psychiatry* 27(4): 447–65.

Surgeon General. 1999. *Mental Health: A Report of the Surgeon General*. Washington: U.S. Department of Health and Human Services.

———. 2001. *Mental Health: Culture, Race, and Ethnicity, A Supplement to Mental Health: A Report of the Surgeon General*. Washington: U.S. Department of Health and Human Services.

Takeuchi, David T., and Sue-Je L. Gage. 2003. "What to Do With Race? Changing Notions of Race in the Social Sciences." In "The Politics of Science: Culture, Race, Ethnicity, and the Supplement to the Surgeon General's Report on Mental Health," edited by Doris F. Chang, Mary-Jo DelVecchio Good, and Byron J. Good. Special issue, *Culture, Medicine and Psychiatry* 27(4): 435–45.

U.S. Census Bureau. Various years. *American FactFinder*. Washington: U.S. Census Bureau. Available at: http://factfinder2.census.gov (accessed May 5, 2010).

Van Ryn, Michelle. 2002. "Research on the Provider Contribution to Race/Ethnicity Disparities in Medical Care." *Medical Care* 40(1): I140–51.

Waters, Mary C. 1999. *Black Identities*. New York: Russell Sage Foundation / Cambridge, Mass.: Harvard University Press.

———. 2008. "Counting and Classifying by Race: The American Debate." *The Tocqueville Review* 29(1): 1–21.

Weinberg, Dana B. 2003. *Code Green*. Ithaca, N.Y.: ILR Press.

Willen, Sarah S., Antonio Bullon, and Mary-Jo DelVecchio Good. 2010. " 'Opening Up a Huge Can of Worms': Reflections on a 'Cultural Sensitivity' Course for Psychiatry Residents." *Harvard Review of Psychiatry* 18(18): 247–53.

Part I

Cultural Environments
of Hyperdiversity

OW ARE health-care institutions responding to the changing demographics, the changing composition of health-care teams, and the increasingly complex configurations of identity that shape the contemporary United States? The four chapters that follow consider both the institutional challenges and the human dilemmas that health-care providers and institutions must confront as they strive to serve an increasingly diverse—and rapidly changing—array of patients and communities. The authors of these chapters, all sociologists and anthropologists, each bring a distinct orientation to this project's core questions. Seth Hannah, a sociologist specializing in inequality, race and ethnic relations, and cultural studies of medicine lends to this collection its hallmark concept of hyperdiversity. Sarah Willen, an anthropologist, approaches Boston's cultural environments through the lens of her ongoing work on how precarious political status and social exclusion can impinge upon immigrants' lived experiences of health, illness, and care-seeking. The anthropologist Lisa Stevenson, who has worked extensively with Inuit, especially on issues of adolescent suicide, considers the limits of human life and the border zones in which possibilities for human engagement are challenged by real or imagined notions of incommensurability.

This part of the volume begins with chapter 2, "Clinical Care in Environments of Hyperdiversity," in which Hannah complicates our understanding of culture by demonstrating the poverty and inadequacy of traditional classificatory schemes—especially the ethnic pentad—within today's hyperdiverse clinical environments. The concept of hyperdiversity is based on the premise that diversity is not just about culture, but can also exist along many dimensions that transcend superficial features, such as phenotype, mother tongue, or nationality. Occasionally culture is blamed within clinical settings as a source of pathology; in other instances, it is regarded by some health-care institutions and providers as a curious flash of the exotic, a frustrating obstacle to diagnosis and treatment, or a problem for someone else—for instance, a medical interpreter, or a hospital chaplain—to manage. Despite these temptations, however, many clinicians are sincerely interested in effectively navigating cultural gaps and finding ways to communicate effectively, and respectfully, with their patients. Hannah reminds us that hyperdiversity is not just about patients. In contemporary cultural environments of hyperdiversity, it is no longer reasonable to presume a dichotomy between "mainstream clinician/ 'Other' patient"; often, these roles are reversed (Willen et al. 2010). As Hannah's analysis reveals, cultural, racial-ethnic, and other forms of diversity, however configured, can serve either as an obstacle to effective care or, if leveraged well, a valuable institutional resource.

As the following three chapters elaborate, many health-care institutions have taken direct action and sought to minimize cultural misunderstandings and improve the quality and effectiveness of patient care. In chapter 3, "Pas de Trois: Medical Interpreters, Clinical Dilemmas, and the Patient-Provider-Interpreter Triad," Sarah Willen considers both the promise and the pitfalls of current efforts to integrate professional interpreters and interpreter service units into health-care teams. Bringing medical interpreters into clinical settings—as mandated by the Commonwealth of Massachusetts and various other states—can prove tremendously useful when patients' limited English proficiency impedes their ability to communicate with care providers and health-care institutions. Significantly, however, both the kind and amount of training interpreters receive vary considerably. Similarly, variation among the models interpreters use to understand the nature and limits of their role is considerable. Are interpreters translating machines or robots who must avoid chit-chat and side conversation, or is theirs a softer role designed to facilitate open, friendly two-way exchange? Ought they focus solely on literal translation, or should they venture beyond the tightly focused patient-care provider dialogue to probe for missing contextual information— cultural, interpersonal, or otherwise—and diagnostic clues? Is the clinical interaction their sole domain of activity, or ought they be empowered— or even required—to work in communities to advocate on patients' behalf? Willen also explores how some clinicians use interpreters as a way of "outsourcing social aspects of the encounter," at times because of their own insecurity or lack of confidence in treating patients across a language barrier. The chapter closes with an instructive observation from several of our interviewees, who note an ironic gap between institutional investment in creating well-staffed, accessible interpreter services, on one hand, and the near-total lack of training for clinicians in working effectively within this new clinical pas de trois.

In chapter 4, "Praying Along: Interfaith Chaplaincy and the Politics of Translation," Stevenson reveals how the nonmedical role of chaplains, like that of medical interpreters, has gained institutional prominence in contemporary environments of hyperdiversity. Whereas health-care institutions tend to regard interpreters as indispensable to the everyday business of clinical care, chaplains and chaplaincy services face a rather different set of constraints. To begin, the chaplain role has been entirely transformed in recent decades from that of the solo, often unpaid lone ranger type to an entirely new model in which chaplains are paid staff members striving for incorporation into the biomedical model of care, including making notes on patients' medical charts (for example, "anointed," followed by initials and date). Stevenson argues that hospitals regard chaplains as providing a cultural service to hospital patients in a way that neutralizes and reworks the potentially divisive matter of religious difference into a tamer form of difference more palatable and comprehensible to hospital bureaucracies. Here it is not any specific religion that hospitals endorse, but rather a culture of religiosity grounded in what Stevenson calls a "universal human need for 'spirituality' in whatever form it takes" or, in Simon Lee's (2002) terms, a black box for patients' psycho-social needs. Religion—or, more precisely, a kind of sanitized or defanged culture of religiosity—is regarded by hospitals as a beneficial and non-threatening way of addressing cultural aspects of patients' illness experiences. Like interpreters, but in different ways, chaplains too are vying for a place within hospital bureaucracies.

Another strategy sometimes used in an effort to bridge cultural difference is clinician-patient matching on the basis of shared cultural or racial-ethnic characteristics. In chapter 5, "Clinician-Patient Matching" Willen notes that in the 1990s, especially following the Surgeon General's 2001 report on disparities in mental health care and the Institute of Medicine's 2003 report, "Unequal Treatment," matching was touted as a way to strengthen clinician-patient rapport and improve outcomes among ethnic-minority patients. A considerable body of subsequent research has cast doubt on these initial assumptions, yet most of these quantitative studies say little about the specific challenges involved in attempting to employ this strategy. The qualitative research design of our study afforded us a unique and illuminating window onto the relative strengths and weaknesses of this technique and, more generally, onto the deep ambivalence with which matching is often regarded by clinicians and patients (see chapters 8 and 9, this volume). The very idea of a match proves complicated given the complex and varied ways in which Americans identify and understand themselves. Who, for instance, would be an appropriate match for President Barack Obama, and why? What if gender, or sexual orientation, provides a more useful basis for matching than culture or race-ethnicity? And what if patients are explicitly opposed—for instance, for reasons of culture or privacy—to consulting a clinician who shares their cultural background? Overall, the clinician interviews we conducted challenge the viability of matching as a strategy for either improving clinician-patient rapport or remediating differences in mental health outcomes, particularly in contemporary cultural environments of hyperdiversity.

References

Lee, Simon J. Craddock. 2002. "In a Secular Spirit: Strategies of Clinical Pastoral Education." *Health Care Analysis* 10: 339–56.

Willen, Sarah S., Antonio Bullon, and Mary-Jo DelVecchio Good. 2010. " 'Opening Up a Huge Can of Worms': Reflections on a 'Cultural Sensitivity' Course for Psychiatry Residents." *Harvard Review of Psychiatry* 18: 247–53.

Chapter 2

Clinical Care in Environments of Hyperdiversity

SETH DONAL HANNAH

TRADITIONALLY home to a rich mix of ethnicities from various European backgrounds and a substantial African American population, Boston has been one of the most diverse and segregated cities in the country. In recent years, however, the nature of this diversity has shifted and become more complex. The loosening of neighborhood residential segregation and new waves of immigration from Latin America, Asia, Africa, and elsewhere have dramatically altered the ethnic landscape. Since 1970, the proportion of nonwhite residents in Suffolk County has increased from 18 to nearly 50 percent, and the number of foreign-born residents from 13 to 28 percent.[1] What is more, increased immigration and ethnic diversity have been accompanied by a geographic redistribution of racial and ethnic groups that has vastly changed the demographic composition of neighborhoods throughout Greater Boston (Allen and Turner 2004). This rapid shift has reconfigured racial and ethnic relations as formerly isolated groups increasingly share residential and community space with other groups (Logan, Oakley, and Stowell 2003; Waters, Ueda, and Marrow 2007; Massey 2008; Bean and Stevens 2003; Bluestone and Stevenson 2000). These changes have the potential both to heighten racial-ethnic tensions and cultural anxieties and to blur the once rigid lines of racial-ethnic classification and boundaries (Waters 1990; Waters, Ueda, and Marrow 2007; Formisano 1991; Wilson and Taub 2006; Alba and Denton 2004; Foner and Fredrickson 2004).[2]

Periods of rapidly increasing diversity are often characterized by a complex interaction among race, ethnicity, immigration, culture, and geographic mobility that has the potential to shift systems of racial and ethnic classification and result in new contours of interpersonal relations (Sundstrom 2003; King 2000). Many scholars are now challenging long-standing notions of race and ethnicity, pointing out that the contemporary system of racial and ethnic classification is a relatively new phenomenon that obscures the historically contingent nature of group boundaries and classifications (Hoschschild and Powell 2008). The system used recently by the U.S. Census Bureau and the National Institutes of Health (NIH) relies on the ethnic pentagon categories of white, black, Asian, Latino, and Native American. Scholars argue that these categories may no longer capture the most salient distinctions between groups (Nobles 2000; Prewitt 2005, 2009; Hattam 2005; Hollinger 1995; Appiah 1996, 2006; Zack 2002; King 2000; Waters 2008).[3] Instead, they suggest that American racial and ethnic relations should be thought of as shifting in a more post-ethnic or cosmopolitan direction.

This chapter investigates this possibility by examining particular social and institutional environments—psychiatric clinics and hospitals—in which broader demographic shifts are manifested. In these settings, patients, doctors, and support staff come together to form a microcosm of racial, ethnic, and cultural interaction. The changing demographic trends seen widely are played out through social interaction in clinical and institutional contexts. In different neighborhoods and cities, each clinic has a particular ethnic-racial-cultural mix that often reflects its surrounding residential environment.

I draw on over 192 interviews with clinical, managerial, and support personnel at psychiatric clinics throughout Greater Boston to examine the way they understand the racial, ethnic, and cultural characteristics of their patient population and how this understanding relates to the census model of the ethnic pentagon. I find that a number of scenarios in clinical settings throughout our study show a racial and ethnic classification system much more complicated than the basic pentagon model implies. Clear boundaries between groups are difficult to discern, and this ambiguity makes it difficult to bind cultural traits with racial and ethnic identity. I introduce and define the concept of hyperdiversity to illustrate these findings.[4]

Racial Classification and Cultural Confusion in Clinical Care

Racial-ethnic diversity in clinical settings can be defined as having a patient population composed of members of easily identifiable racial or ethnic groups as defined by the ethnic pentagon (Hollinger 1995; Hochschild and Powell 2008; Waters 2008). This formulation, which has its roots in the civil rights movement and the period of liberalized immigration policies after 1965, blends the long-standing black-white divide with the pan-ethnicity movements that have emerged since the civil rights era (King 2000; Winant 2000).[5] The pan-ethnic categories of Asian American and Hispanic mirrored the group-based solidarity of racial identity politics by unifying disparate cultural and immigrant groups under the banner of a single identity category as a way to express their common interests (Bean and Tienda 1987; Sommers 1991; Espiritu 1992; Lopez and Espiritu 1997). As a result, within-group differences were subsumed to mobilize against a common external threat: racial- or ethnic-based discrimination in the United States. These pan-ethnic identity categories have attained broad popular acceptance. In the case of Asian Americans, the strength of the pan-ethnic category was reinforced by shared racial group ascription, whereas with Hispanics/Latinos, it was bolstered by shared language and religious orientation. This helped the Hispanic/Latino category cohere, even though its members can technically be of any race (Lopez and Espiritu 1997).[6]

The salience of these categories has had a tremendous impact on health-care institutions in recent decades as decreasing residential segregation and increased immigration have raised the likelihood of multiple racial-ethnic groups being seen at a given clinic site. Clinicians and staff accustomed to practicing in a much more monolithic racial-ethnic environment have faced new challenges as their patient populations have grown more diverse.

Chief among these challenges were the various cultural differences that emerged as important in the process of delivering care. As medical anthropologists pointed out, behavior, disease manifestations, and communication vary across racial and ethnic populations (Kleinman 1980; Good 1977, 1994; Nichter 1981; Kleinman, Eisenberg, and Good 1978; Good and Good 1980, 1981; Good et al. 2003). A large body of literature has emerged documenting the ways in which cultural differences challenge standard models of practice and the consequences that stem from not adjusting to them, namely, health disparities and unequal treatment (Smedley, Stith, and Nelson 2003). For example, Stanley Sue describes the problem as

> the inadequacy of services for members of ethnic minority groups such as African Americans, American Indians, Asian Americans, and Hispanics/Latinos. One of the most frequently cited problems in delivering mental health services to ethnic minority groups is the cultural and linguistic mismatches that occur between clients and providers. Cultural differences can affect the validity of assessment as well as the development of therapist-client rapport, the therapeutic alliance, and treatment effectiveness. (Sue 1998, 441)

Such sentiments have led to the development of new legal frameworks, manuals, teaching guidelines for medical students, and culturally specific treatment protocols (Betancourt et al. 2003; Lakes, Lopez, and Garro 2006; Brach and Fraser 2000; Sue 1998; Lo and Stacey 2008). Many of these programs associate cultural traits with ethnic group membership in an effort to teach health-care providers about the cultural characteristics of their patients (Flores, Gee, and Kastner 2000; Vega 2005; Lo and Stacey 2008).[7] It is not uncommon to find treatment manuals or training sessions instructing clinicians that Asian patients may be family oriented, that Middle Eastern women will prefer being examined by women, or that post-traumatic stress disorder (PTSD) has different manifestations in African Americans than it does in Asians, whites, or Hispanics/Latinos (Pole, Gone, and Kulkarni 2008).

The key underlying assumption is that providers can recognize the ethnic group membership of their patients and tailor care in keeping with the cultural characteristics associated with that particular group (Guarnaccia, Vega, and Bonner 2006; Kagawa-Singer and Kassim-Lakha 2003; Guarnaccia and Rodriguez 1996; see also Fox 1995; Shaw 2005; Taylor 2003). They treat racial and ethnic identity as a proxy for underlying cultural characteristics that are thought to impact health, help-seeking behaviors, and quality of care (Kirmayer and Sartorius 2007; Hunt 2005). Culture is often seen as pathological; a barrier to be overcome if optimal care is to be provided. Treatment manuals and training programs seek to overcome these barriers by educating clinicians and support staff about problematic cultural factors on a group-by-group basis (Santiago-Irizarry 2001; Borovoy and Hine 2008).[8]

Although it is clear that cultural diversity often covaries with racial and ethnic classifications, it does not necessarily always do so. Cultural diversity can exist within ethnic groups as well, and other dimensions of culture (such as those deriving from class background or education) do not cleanly match up with ethnic identity (Ford 2008; Kim et al. 2001). This has led some respondents in our study to question the crude association of cultural traits to broad groups of patients. As Mary, an interfaith chaplain who works with inpatient psychiatric patients, explained, "I can't ever know what the other person's really like—I have to find out, and just because this is an African American patient or student doesn't mean that they're exactly like the list says they are."

Several clinicians we interviewed wrestled with the question of how information about the cultural traits generally associated with different racial or ethnic groups should be used to determine and understand the cultural traits of individual patients. For example, Dr. Romanak, a male psychiatry resident at a large academic hospital, suggested that he would prefer an expanded approach to determining whether cultural difference is relevant to a case—one that goes beyond simplistic group-based treatment protocols. When I asked him about his personal approach to treating diverse patients, he responded,

It's important . . . for me to learn as much as I can from the patient and from collateral information. . . . I think protocols in general are just bad, that it's always better to try to cater specifically to whoever you're dealing with. I find that when you're dealing with cultures that are different than your own, it takes a lot more work and asking more questions and going to different sources in order to parse it out and make sense of it in your mind.

Instead of relying solely on group-based treatment protocols that instruct appropriate treatment for patients of different ethnic backgrounds, Romanak spends additional time probing the patient and seeks out additional information from other members of the treatment team. These collateral sources may have more knowledge about the cultural norms of ethnic groups he is unfamiliar with. For example, when treating a Japanese woman who presented to the emergency room with "a kind of psychotic paranoia," Romanak consulted with her language teacher, who told him she was behaving in ways that even the Japanese students in the class recognized as not being culturally normal for a Japanese woman her age. He also sought cultural advice from the Japanese interpreter as well as her English-speaking family members. In short, Romanak was relying on the advice of what have been described as "cultural brokers," who helped bridge the gap of cultural difference (Geertz 1960; Lo 2010).

Dr. Desmond, a senior psychiatrist at the same large academic hospital, also exemplified this approach, calling for a mix of individual exploration and the use of cultural brokers. However, he calls attention to the issue of time constraint, which limits his ability to elicit cultural information directly from his patients. When I asked him whether he has any particular strategies for dealing with patients from different racial-ethnic backgrounds, given time constraints, he replied, "Hopefully you have more than just a little bit of a window, because if there is only a little window, it's hard to get to that—just the more you can communicate with somebody and talk to them, and try and figure out where they're coming from and how they're viewing what's going on."

Desmond is suggesting here that if given enough time to communicate with the patient, he may be able to figure out whether there are any important cultural factors involved. However, he does not see this as ideal. Instead, he seeks outside counsel from someone culturally similar to the patient to make sure there's not something he's missing:

The ideal situation would be if you see someone from a different cultural background, meet with them, and you have another clinician around from that same background who you can talk to and find out if there's something you're missing in the way this person is viewing the situation. So, sometimes you can do that. It's not always available.

When seeking additional insight about potential cultural factors, Desmond turns to others from that same background for help, relying on another clinician, an interpreter, a clerical staff member, or even a family member to explain "why the person may be viewing something in a certain way."[9] This reflects the theory of explanatory models that underlies how cultural issues are often understood in the contemporary culture of medicine (Kleinman, Eisenberg, and Good 1978). Both Desmond and Romanak view cultural differences in the way patients understand their illness and experience as an important factor to consider in their daily work. However, by seeking the advice of cultural brokers or others who share the cultural identity of the patient, they do so in a way that uses identity as a proxy for culture.

Hyperdiversity and the Breakdown of Racial-Ethnic Identity As Cultural Proxy

The use of identity as a proxy for culture makes sense when the link between the two is strong. But what happens when the link breaks down? If clinicians and support staff are operating on the assumption that racial or ethnic group membership is coherent and persistent and that members of these groups share a bundle of relevant cultural characteristics, they may treat patients differently on the basis of that assumption. This works fine as long as the cultural assumption is accurate. When it is not, inappropriate stereotyping, misdiagnosis, and mistrust can occur. One classic case is the overdiagnosis of black males with schizophrenia (Good et al. 2003; Metzl 2010). Research shows that psychiatrists have historically been more likely to diagnose black males with schizophrenia based on assumptions about the cultural characteristics of black patients—that they are more prone to violence (Metzl 2010).

Closely linking identity to cultural characteristics can also have an impact on the treatment experience. For example, clinicians often assume that psychotherapy patients prefer to be treated by clinicians that are racially or ethnically similar to themselves. However, recent research has found that a significant minority of patients, particularly recent immigrants and refugees, do not prefer ethnically similar clinicians for fear that their personal information will leak to members of their community. What is more, despite common sense notions that matching is effective, the preponderance of evidence from peer-reviewed studies does not show positive effects (Maramba and Hall 2002; Shin et al. 2005; chapter 3, this volume; see also Chang and Berk 2009).

Another example is the assumption that medication noncompliance varies across ethnic groups systematically because of cultural differences.

Recent studies have found that psychiatrists will tailor their choice of medication to prescribe for a patient depending on the patient's anticipated likelihood to properly maintain the regimen. Latino patients are often singled out as having negative attitudes toward medications and are prescribed older medications with simpler dosing that may be less effective (Smedley, Stith, and Nelson 2003; Ng et al. 1996). Moreover, whether clinicians make cultural assumptions based on identity is highly consequential; it can mean the difference between a proper and improper diagnosis, a positive or negative therapeutic alliance between a client and a therapist, or the successful or unsuccessful dosing of a medication.

I now turn to discuss the way racial, ethnic, and cultural boundaries were constructed and understood in our various clinical sites in greater Boston—both by patients themselves and by clinicians and staff. I found that patients, clinicians, and staff were not easily classified according to the U.S. Census– and NIH-based racial and ethnic categories of the ethnic pentagon. This disrupted clinicians' efforts to use identity as a proxy for cultural characteristics when trying to address cultural issues in clinical interactions. As a result, clinicians often viewed the importance of culture in ways that had little to do with broad racial and ethnic classifications; instead, they focused on issues of language, immigration status, and nationality, and on nonethnic forms of cultural difference, such as socioeconomic class and illness category.

I developed the concept of hyperdiversity to describe these findings and as a general way to describe social environments where similar conditions exist. I refer to these as cultural environments of hyperdiversity. A cultural environment of hyperdiversity is a social setting that is *highly diverse* (in terms of race and ethnicity as well as social class, immigration status and religion), *dynamic* (unstable or undergoing change), and *multidimensional* (individuals may choose to identify with broad racial and ethnic categories or narrower categories such as country of origin, neighborhood, or sexual orientation). In these settings, racial and ethnic classification is more difficult, and the link between census-based racial and ethnic identities and culture is likely to be weak or broken (shattered). Moreover, the concept of hyperdiversity encourages us to think more broadly about diversity and the forms of difference that are likely to be salient in a given social setting. Race and ethnicity may not be the most dominant forms of social identity as other contextually dependent patterns of social categorization emerge.

I illustrate the concept of hyperdiversity by discussing five scenarios we observed in our Greater Boston field sites. In these five scenarios, the application of a coherent racial-ethnic classification structure to take culture into account in the provision of care was disrupted, revealing the complexity of applying the standard cultural sensitivity approach to care. The scenarios are as follows:

- *multiplicity,* where the sheer number of different racial-ethnic groups makes organizing services based on identity impractical;

- *ambiguity,* where a patient's racial-ethnic group membership is not easily labeled or understood using physical features alone;

- *simultaneity,* where labeling is difficult because individuals occupy multiple racial-ethnic categories at once;

- *fluidity,* where labeling is difficult because of the flexibility and fluidity of a patient's self-asserted racial or ethnic identity; and

- *misapplication,* where an individual's racial-ethnic group membership is correctly identified but the individual fails to share significant cultural characteristics with that group.

These scenarios reveal a complex environment in which modern medicine struggles to provide equitable, high quality care in a way that both recognizes the reality of culturally based disparities and seeks to avoid reproducing them.

Settings of Hyperdiversity

The ecological characteristics of hyperdiversity were particularly present in two of our clinical field sites: Neighborhood Community Health Center (NCHC) and Private Psychiatric Hospital (PPH). Both are located in communities experiencing high rates of immigration and rapid change in their racial and ethnic demographics. I describe the racial, ethnic, and linguistic diversity at these clinics and elaborate the five scenarios of hyperdiversity.

Neighborhood Community Health Center

At NCHC, a large community health-care center in a dense lower-income urban community outside Boston, Spanish-speaking patients make up nearly 70 percent of the patient population, mostly recent immigrants from Central and South America. This population has grown rapidly in recent years. Between 2000 and 2004, the numbers of Salvadorans increased 66 percent, Colombians 96 percent, Hondurans 135 percent, and Guatemalans 159 percent (Shea and Jones 2006). Before 1990, however, immigrants from these countries were nearly nonexistent in this community, and the majority of patients at NCHC were Irish, Italian, Polish, Russian, and African American.[10] Today, these groups make up less than 20 percent of the population.

The ethnic composition has shifted so fast that when the health center was constructed in 1999, a significant number of Vietnamese patients were projected to patronize the facility, and all signs in the building were written in English, Spanish, and Vietnamese. Today, Vietnamese patients are rarely seen, and no Vietnamese interpreters or clinicians are on staff. What is more, although Spanish-speaking patients currently make up the majority of patients at the health center, the range of ethnic and linguistic diversity among the remaining mix of patients is remarkable. NCHC is located in a refugee resettlement area. It has provided care for successive waves of refugees first from the former Yugoslavian territories during the 1990s and from a variety of African and Middle Eastern countries in the 2000s, including more than 500 Bantus from Somalia. Approximately 33,000 people—speaking thirty languages—live in a 1.5-square-mile area surrounding the health center.

Over the last decade, as the Spanish-speaking population grew, the health center gradually filled a significant proportion of clinical and support positions with native and non-native Spanish speakers. Approximately 30 percent of the patients at NCHC speak only Spanish, and another 30 percent are bilingual Spanish-English speakers. Nearly all front desk and clerical workers speak Spanish fluently, but only half of the social workers, nurses, and doctors do. This leaves NCHC better equipped than most to handle the needs of Spanish-speaking patients, but they are always looking to add capacity. The two most common complaints I heard from staff were that there were not enough Spanish-language interpreters and that it was impossible to find Spanish-speaking psychiatrists.

Private Psychiatric Hospital

Ward B is twenty-six-bed inpatient psychiatric unit for adults with acute mental illness and is located within Private Psychiatric Hospital, a private, for-profit facility. PPH has a policy of taking the most severely ill patients that other treatment programs refuse to take, and over the years it has become a refuge for the most disadvantaged and difficult patients in the Boston area. Because of its location in inner-city Boston, PPH has a high concentration of lower-income black and Hispanic/Latino patients. Although approximately 40 percent of patients on the unit at any given time might be identified by others as racially black, they are also a diverse mix of recent immigrants or second- and third-generation Americans from the Dominican Republic, Haiti, Puerto Rico, the West Indies, or Cape Verde—as well as multiple-generation African Americans.[11] What is more, a majority are more likely to self-identify ethnically based on their country of origin than as black or African American. The staff is similarly approximately 40 percent black, but though the black patients are largely American-born or immigrants from the Caribbean, the majority of the black staff—including the unit manager—are immigrants from Nigeria (often students or recent college graduates with an interest in mental health). The Nigerian staff, who aside from the manager fill the lower-level jobs on the unit, only recently learned about the history of racism toward black Americans (and especially the Tuskegee episode) and do not feel culturally similar to them.[12]

Hispanics and Latinos, who make up 30 percent of the patients and 10 percent of staff at PPH, have similarly diverse backgrounds—most being from Puerto Rico or the Dominican Republic. With a full-time Spanish-speaking psychiatrist and psychologist on staff, Ward B is nominally known as a Latino unit and attracts Spanish-speaking patients from as far away as Springfield, Brockton, and Lawrence, Massachusetts. Compared with the Hispanic/Latino patients at NCHC, the Hispanics and Latinos on Ward B at PPH are more likely to have mixed racial background, be bilingual, and speak primarily English. The bilingual patients are given the option to see the Spanish-speaking psychiatrist and to attend group sessions with the Spanish-speaking therapist. Patients with limited English ability tend to attend Spanish-speaking groups and do not interact much with others on the unit, including the bilingual patients. The bilingual patients rarely choose the Spanish groups and thus are fully integrated with the rest of the unit. The remaining 30 percent of patients identify racially as white, a majority of whom identify ethnically as Irish, Italian American, or mixed European ancestry.

Scenarios of Hyperdiversity

In settings of hyperdiversity, the relationship between race, ethnicity, and culture is likely to be complex. During field research, I observed five scenarios—multiplicity, ambiguity, simultaneity, fluidity, and misapplication—that illustrate problems with racial and ethnic classification and with associating cultural characteristics with racial or ethnic identity.

Multiplicity

Multiplicity occurs in settings like these, where there is such a high level of racial-ethnic diversity that dividing and organizing services based on identity dimensions is impractical or simply doesn't make sense. In this circumstance, patients may be members of identity groups that are easily labeled and understood, but staff capacity is not enough to address the unique aspects of each group. The outpatient mental health department at NCHC, which is affiliated with a large academic medical center, regularly treats patients who speak thirteen languages. The health center simply does not have the resources available to its patron hospital to accommodate this level of linguistic diversity. It is financially prohibitive to employ interpreters for each language, much less cultural specialists who could provide insight on how cultural background may impact patients' health and health care. Dr. Berry, the corporate manager of psychiatry for the large health-care network that administers NCHC, summarized this problem well. Explaining his approach to cultural issues, he said,

> different cultures are going to have different concepts about what it means to get psychotherapy and/or to be on medication . . . if someone is of Asian descent and specifically say they're Korean or Vietnamese or Cambodian, or if they're of African descent and they're from Nigeria or Ethiopia, you really have to understand in a cultural context what their meaning of getting help is, in particular psychiatric help, and I think that to not understand that is to really miss the boat in terms of being somebody who could then work with somebody from that culture if they're not of that culture. And again I don't think there's enough providers in the state of Massachusetts to provide in a cultural context to a particular immigrant group.

Berry underscores the importance of understanding, in cultural context, the meaning that patients place on getting help and views these cultural differences as existing across multiple levels of identity (for Asians and Africans and for national subgroups within them such as Korean or Nigerian). According to Berry, to not understand this is to miss the boat in terms of being able to work cross-culturally. This suggests that to be sensitive to these differences would require an individual clinician to be familiar with the cultural meanings of each conceivable group or would require hiring someone from that culture for each group. As Berry explains, there are not enough providers in the state of Massachusetts to accomplish this goal. Finding clinicians and support staff who share the racial background of the patient is impractical enough, but considering the wide range of cultural diversity within racial groups only amplifies the problem. Under this logic, the number of cultural aggregations to be accounted for is infinite.

In clinics where patients from a particular cultural background are numerous, it may be possible to maintain staff who are familiar with or share that background. But where no one group dominates and the demographic mix of patients frequently shifts, it is more difficult for staff demographics to closely match that of the patients. At NCHC, in addition to improving Spanish-language services, management constantly monitors the changing demographics to ensure that support systems are in place as new groups enter the area. Although they can draw on local Spanish-speaking residents who have lived in the area for some time to fill these positions, it is much more difficult to accommodate the variety of newly arriving immigrant groups with other language needs. As Pamela, director of community and refugee health told me, "It's really, what do we need to do specially to target them to make them feel welcome here? The kind of ramping up of new services or staff really has much more to do with new people that are coming rather than the folks that have lived here for a long time."

Although the health center tries to ramp up services for new arrivals, it is frustrated by hiring rules that require new employees to be credentialed in the United States. This becomes a problem when it wishes to hire or promote capable staff who earned degrees from another countries or have proved themselves qualified beyond their credentials. As Pamela explains,

> Ever since I came here I've fundamentally believed that it's a very diverse team that's able to do the work the best, so I've always looked to hire people from the countries of the patients that we're serving to try and facilitate the work. And that's been a real uphill battle because somebody from Somalia might not have their degree from here but they might be incredibly qualified. So our system is set up to say, "Well you know, you have to have your degree from here, you have to have your work experience from here," so I feel like I've always pushed against systems and boundaries and rules to try and create the team that I've created. Several years back—the community health team keeps growing—there was a commitment to say should there be an assistant director of the community health team. And the thought from other folks was, "Let's hire somebody from outside and bring them in to help," and my push back was, "No, let me take some of my staff who are incredibly qualified and talented here and let me try and mentor them and give them the opportunity to grow into managers themselves."

Pamela has had some success hiring and mentoring non-traditional candidates to build a diverse staff, but she has had to "push against systems" to do it. Furthermore, these efforts bear fruit only when the particular group constitutes a meaningful portion of the patient population. When a significant group leaves the area and no longer requires services, the staff recruited and mentored into these positions need to be phased out, forcing management to repeat the process. As Pamela says, "What's hard is when folks move out. When I first came we had a Vietnamese interpreter. Over time the Vietnamese population has moved out of (the area). There's very few left. What's hard for me is that then I have a staff person that I have to sort of downsize or see whether there's a way to roll them into another position."

At NCHC, the patient population is incredibly diverse and constantly shifting. Management actively monitors these changes and seeks to build new capacity when new groups arrive and others leave. However, these efforts are challenged by hiring rules, the sheer numbers of different groups, and their instability.

Racial Ambiguity

In contrast to situations of multiplicity, when readily defined groups are numerous, situations also exist in which the racial-ethnic group membership of the patients is not easily labeled or understood by staff.

This happens when individuals are racially ambiguous—that is, their phenotype is such that they are not easily lumped into one of the major racial groups commonly employed in the United States. This most often occurs when people are of mixed heritage, and is especially common among patients from Latin America, particularly the Caribbean or Brazil. At PPH so much ambiguity surrounds the racial identity of patients, the staff ask each other about the identity of certain patients. When I asked Mary, an Irish American nurse, about the racial identity of the patients she sees, she responded, "There's been times that I've been asked, is a person, is he black, white, whatever; and there's times when I actually can't say. And I've noticed that more, I don't know if it's a fact that people are more mixed or if it's just, I don't know, you get to know the person and you kind of forget that identifying characteristic, but I was just going to say we have people that are a combination of races and ethnicities."

The patient population at PPH is racially and ethnically diverse. PPH sees the largest number of Caribbean patients, particularly Puerto Ricans and Dominicans, of any Boston-area hospital.[13] These patients do not appear phenotypically white or black, and when asked about their racial identity, nearly all choose to identify themselves as Puerto Ricans or Dominicans (nationality), or as Latino or Spanish (pan-ethnic). They rarely use the racial labels white, black, or mixed to describe themselves. This matches the results from the 2000 U.S. Census, showing that the majority of respondents choosing Other as their racial category also chose Hispanic/Latino as their ethnicity (see also Roth 2006).

In casual conversations with staff members, I asked how they perceived the racial diversity of the patient population. The answer I received became a common refrain, "It's mixed, it's just very mixed!" As I explored the issue further, instead of getting a detailed list of the racial and ethnic characteristics of the population, I would instead receive in-depth descriptions of language usage and illness categories. Raymond, an Eastern European–born, American-raised group therapist on one of the acute inpatient psychiatric units, said this when asked about the racial-ethnic characteristics of his patients:

> Raymond: So, there's quite a mix. In terms of the ethnicity, the two major ethnic groups that we have are—with *ethnicity,* what do you mean by *ethnicity?* Where people come from?
>
> Q: Whatever. How do you understand it?
>
> Raymond: How do I understand it? Fine. So, my immediate thought is where people come from, which is mainly the language they speak because I sort of emphasize the language in my work, how much people can verbalize their impulses, so I'm thinking Spanish-speaking patients and English-speaking patients. We also have a division in terms of race.

> We have black people and white people and we have quite a division in terms of age. We certainly have division in terms of gender. In terms of age we take patients from eighteen to however old they are and there's a clear division in terms of gender, which is obvious. In terms of anything, the main one is between Spanish and English speaking.

The group therapist was initially confused by the question, and when given the flexibility to define it for himself, decided to frame the issue mainly in terms of language rather than ethnicity. Acknowledging that there are racial divisions on the unit, he went on to note that 70 percent of the patient population speaks English only and nearly 30 percent speak Spanish (half of whom have limited English proficiency, the other half bilingual but preferring to be treated by English speakers). When asked if it was relatively easy for him to understand who among his patients is what racial-ethnic group, he responded,

> Raymond: I guess not because when you asked me I had a problem even with the idea of what do you mean by ethnicity. I guess I don't think about it in my daily work. I do think of it in terms of language.
>
> Q: Why don't you think about it in terms of your daily work?
>
> Raymond: Well, I only think of it in terms of language because I'm coming into work thinking how am I going to find a way to communicate with these people. So, my emphasis is on—when I approach a person I am more interested in what language they speak than where they are from.

This case underscores the widely held view among clinicians and staff at PPH that language is one of the most important group-level phenomena they face on a daily basis, one which vastly overshadows issues related to race.

This was definitely the case with Spanish-speaking patients at PPH. Ward B has enough Spanish-language capacity among the staff to make it a destination for Spanish-speaking psychiatric patients in need of short-term hospitalization. The unit is described as having a Latino program, yet there is great consternation among the staff that they do not provide rich layers of services in Spanish. The twenty-six-bed unit has a Spanish-speaking psychiatrist and social worker, along with two Spanish-speaking mental health associates, in addition to numerous non-Spanish-speaking support staff. Yet they do not currently have a Spanish-speaking nurse and only offer irregularly scheduled group therapy sessions for Spanish speakers. What is more, these efforts are seen as basic language accommodation— not culturally sensitive care. The staff jokingly refers to moving an extra television set into a conference room so that patients can view Spanish-language television in the evenings as the most meaningful service they provide to Spanish-speaking patients.

The opinion of the staff members I spoke with is that up to 50 percent of the patients on any given day are Hispanic, Latino, or Spanish—terms that staffers use interchangeably. They list a number of countries of origin, and recognize that racial backgrounds often vary and are mixed. However, little attention is paid to the particularities of the background of Spanish-speaking patients on the unit, and no effort is made to culturally tailor treatment to Spanish-speaking patients, either on the basis of Hispanic/Latino identity or on more narrow categorical bases. When I asked Raya, a young, newly minted nurse of South Asian descent, if country of origin mattered for Hispanic/Latino patients on the unit, she responded, "No . . . not really . . . like occasionally I happen to know just because we write it on the maps. The nurses do the admission paperwork so, you know, we'll put their country of origin in there. A lot of people I don't think even know the country of origin. Patients know because a lot of the Puerto Ricans will stick together or, you know, the Dominicans will stick together. So we know that way but I don't think I ever paid attention."

Instead, language is considered the key force that binds the Hispanic/Latino population together in the eyes of staff. Mary, whose views are broadly representative of other staff on the unit, considers the Spanish-speaking patients on the unit to be from widely diverse racial and cultural backgrounds, which makes cultural targeting an unviable approach. As she explains,

> because we have to market to many Spanish-speaking patients from the various countries, I think to try to group them into one cultural background and say, "Oh, we want to focus on their Spanish culture," that's not really possible because these people are coming from many different cultures. If at least we can try to meet the language as a first language and not try to hear from them through a translator, I think it's very, very helpful. To try to address every one of these cultures or to try to group people into like, "Oh they're all Latino, so of course therefore they're like this," I think that's unrealistic.

This section illustrates a clinical environment in which the racial-ethnic group membership of the patients is not easily labeled or considered relevant by staff. Clinical and support staff view race, ethnicity, and culture as a messy mix and resist delving into the cultural intricacies of particular racial and ethnic groups. Instead, patient categorization is usually made according to language.

Simultaneity

Situations where labeling is difficult also occur when individuals occupy multiple racial-ethnic categories at once. This makes it challenging for providers to determine which is the most relevant classification. This occurs when, for example, a phenotypically black patient is also an immigrant or refugee from a particular country in Africa. While racially black, this person may have had no exposure to American society and comes from a different cultural context than a phenotypically black person who is an American descendant of some mixture of white and African ancestry.

Recent research has shown that in places like New York City, where African Americans and West Indians share residential space and compete in the labor market, employers have become keenly aware of the cultural differences between the two groups. In her book *Black Identities*, Mary Waters found that some employers have developed stereotypical perceptions of black Americans as less desirable workers than West Indians on the basis of what they perceive as a weaker work ethic and less friendly disposition on the job (1999). When she interviewed West Indian immigrants, they argued that they and other West Indians like them merited inclusion in American society because of their strong work ethic, emphasis on education, and lack of pathological behaviors. According to Waters, "by asserting an immigrant or an ethnic identity, West Indians can make a case that they are culturally different from black Americans" (342).

Distinctions between West Indians and American blacks were found to be very important in our study. At Academic Medical Center 1 (AMC1) in Boston, for example, although the numbers of black and West Indian patients are not large, those of blacks and West Indians employed in service-level staff positions throughout the hospital are. Here, as with the West Indians in New York City (Waters 1999), black employees from Jamaica or Trinidad and Tobago (partly in response to real or potential racial discrimination) tend to downplay their racial identities as black Americans and instead play up their immigrant identity and the cultural differences that go along with it. Angela, a forty-year-old West Indian operations manager on the inpatient unit at AMC1 captured this dynamic well in her discussion with me:

Q: And do you feel like people think of you as being from West Indies and being an immigrant, or do you think people see you as a black woman? Do you feel like because of your identity that there's any sort of tension there between people looking at you as an immigrant?

Angela: No. Personally, I think the fact that I'm an immigrant stands out, and if you don't know me, and you haven't heard me speak, then I think the first perception is, "There's an African American." And it probably don't even make them stand back, until I open my mouth and they realize, "Oh she has a strong accent." Some people look at the way I dress and some people say, "That's a West Indian color!" And I'm like, "What's a West Indian color?"

Q: The fact that it's color?

Angela: Yes, bright colors. Bright colors, but you just get past these things. I can go on and on. One woman asked me, what did I use to comb my hair, on my unit, and I wanted to slap her, because I thought you couldn't be more stupid. But I also thought, it's not just me, and she wasn't trying to be stupid.

Q: She just didn't know. I also wanted to ask this question about this difference between being black and being an immigrant.

Angela: That probably has to do with individual experiences and interaction with a particular group. Sometimes they look at you and they may tend to stereotype a particular group or each person from that particular group in that manner. And you're absolutely right. That's one of the reasons that I'm always reminded, and I do tell people I'm first an immigrant, I'm first a West Indian. And when they can differentiate between Trinidad and Jamaica, that's fine, and some people cannot. Some people are offended and they make a big deal.

These comments illustrate the distinctions that exist for individuals who simultaneously occupy multiple racial-ethnic-cultural positions. The people in Angela's workplace attempt to classify her first as an African American—using racial identity as the primary factor—even though she sees herself primarily as a member of a distinct cultural or immigrant group. In response, Angela resists this labeling by asserting a strong ethnic and cultural identity as a West Indian.

Although rarely physicians, black West Indians are employed extensively throughout the hospital as vocational nurses, dietary specialists, and custodial workers. In this capacity, they are in direct day-to-day interactions with patients. When staff is composed of black West Indians from different islands, conflicts can arise between them over the perceived quality of care being given to patients on the units. I asked how this affects patient care when the nursing staff and physicians are unaware of these nuances:

Angela: It does not interfere with patient care from that level, but it does at the lower level, at the base level. Here you have more interaction with the diverse minority groups at the higher levels. There are very few West Indians in the higher groups, at the nursing level, compared to [cleaning staff]. Right. Most of the West Indian staff are dietary or cleaning staff, whether they are West Indian or from a minority group. The conflict comes in with staff. Because if you have two people working on the same unit, just they're both minorities, you think they will be friends and get along, and it doesn't always happen.

Q: So there's interpersonal conflict.

Angela: And sometimes it interferes. However, it affects patient care in if I'm cleaning, I'm Trinidadian, there's another woman from Trinidad in the bed, I will go above and beyond to make sure that room is sparkling. She may need something from dietary; she may want something else instead of orange juice. She may like blend, then I will go above and beyond to do these little things and just make that patient a little more comfortable. And you may not extend yourself quite as well for, let's say, a Jamaican.

Instead of confirming my suggestion that lack of awareness by staff (especially management) of ethnic differences might present problems, Angela states that in her experience, the opposite occurs. Diversity presents more problems for administrative staff involved in direct patient care and involves heightened awareness of ethnic difference rather than unawareness. Dietary workers she supervised often favored patients who shared their ethnic background. I asked her whether, from a managerial perspective, she thinks that such behavior is legitimate or something she would encourage.

Angela: I would definitely not encourage that. And on this unit, we're fortunate that two people who actually have to work together, they're from the Cape Verde islands, so they're friendly. From the Cape culture they get along well, they can just do what they like. They also treat the Cape Verdean patients differently. There's a lot more interaction, like they were going, for example, and they would braid the hair of the patient. Otherwise they would not do it.

Q: How can they have that much time? That's crazy!

Angela: But they do that, and they may do that for someone else in another minority group, because it's someone who looks like them, so they can relate, they can sympathize.

Angela does not condone ethnic favoritism by staff. However, she complicates the matter by suggesting that it sometimes can work well for the patients and staff involved. She also suggests that favoritism can at times extend beyond narrow ethnic group membership to include "someone who looks like them." This seems to imply that racial group membership can also form the basis of connection between staff and patients. Similar to other minority groups with significant African ancestry such as African Americans, West Indians, and Hispanics/Latinos, Cape Verdeans commonly keep their hair in braids. According to Angela, this can form a basis of solidarity between staff and patients who share these characteristics.

This exchange highlights the complexity that exists when clinical environments are composed of individuals who occupy multiple racial-ethnic-cultural categories at once. The divide between American blacks and West Indians, and even among West Indians, can shape the process of care in small and unexpected ways. Staff diversity can be as important as patient diversity in shaping the social environment of the clinic. Despite the potential for differential treatment, interpersonal conflicts, and other difficulties, there is also potential for increased sympathy and understanding. The complexity of these relationships provides both challenges and opportunities for organizations in hyperdiverse environments.

This complexity is also evident at PPH, where immigrants from Nigeria make up nearly a third of the workforce on Ward B, including the unit manager and over half of the mental health associates. The Nigerian Americans working on Ward B self-identify racially as black or African and are viewed as such by patients and other staff members on the unit. This said, they also and simultaneously occupy other identity categories that shape their experience on the unit. Their interactions with patients and coworkers are shaped by their nationality as Nigerians, their ethno-linguistic background as either Igbo or Yoruba, their status as recent immigrants, as well as their black racial identity.

In staff interviews, many of these cultural differences are illustrated. One of the most prominent differences concerns views of the nature of mental illness. Some of the Nigerians do not see mental illness as being a biologically based medical problem, but look instead to supernatural explanations such as curses and spirits. Bernard, the highly respected forty-five-year-old Nigerian-born manager of Ward B, discussed with me how mental illness is viewed in Nigeria, and also his own views of mental illness and how they have evolved since immigrating to America.

> Well, it started changing when I started first working here and I actually saw that people were being admitted to hospital for depression or for suicidal thoughts and sometimes even for drug use. And because in Nigeria when I was growing up, you couldn't tell anyone that you were thinking about killing yourself. I mean, it just, people, it's a sign of weakness. You just wouldn't share with people because you'd be considered physically weak or people would basically shun you. It wasn't anything that you could do, you're supposed to reach out to family, you're supposed to be strong.

Bernard is suggesting that in Nigeria, suicidal ideation is constructed as an individual, private matter that people are supposed to deal with on their own. Seeking treatment or admitting problems is seen as a sign of weakness. Drug abuse, a common cause for hospitalization at PPH, is also seen much differently in Nigeria. Bernard describes it as follows: "In terms of drug use, if you went to a hospital in Nigeria and said, "I want to be hospitalized, I was using drugs," they will arrest you and send you to the police. And also, sort of like a social shame that sort of goes along with saying that you do things that society don't approve, like drug use."

Bernard suggests that not only are aspects of mental illness considered a private matter and a sign of weakness in Nigeria, but they can also be seen as deviant and worthy of criminal punishment and imprisonment. To the extent that psychiatric treatment facilities exist in Nigeria, as Bernard asserts, they serve very few, leaving most of the mentally ill to live on the streets (for the history of psychiatry in Nigeria, see Lambo 1956).[14] According to Bernard,

> schizophrenia, which deals with hallucinations, these are things that, as I said, people just leave in the street. When I went to the cities in Nigeria I knew that psychiatric hospitals exist, but I didn't know what they do. It was nothing that I had read about, so the whole thing with mental illness is that it is just considered something that is not curable, you can't really do anything about it. And I guess in Nigerian society we don't really pay attention to it.

On arriving in the United States and gaining exposure to the American approach, he began to view what he considered the Nigerian approach as too austere. He sought to bring a much more empathetic, personal approach to his own work as manager of the acute inpatient unit at PPH. However, his views are influenced by the fact he comes from a very educated and well-read and well-traveled family, and he notes that other African staff members do not necessarily share his approach. In fact, although Bernard has always rejected supernatural explanations of mental illness, at least two Nigerian mental health associates I interviewed acknowledged that they still question the biological basis of mental illness, even after living in the United States for some time and working on an inpatient psychiatric unit. Many others, though clearly adopting a biological understanding of mental illness, were still influenced by Nigerian norms toward the mentally ill. They were often skeptical of the severity of patients' conditions and questioned patients' need for treatment.

During my field work, a consensus view emerged among the staff and patients that black African staff generally have a more stern and strict approach to patient care when compared with the other mental health associates. Other mental health associates and nurses criticize this approach for impeding the development of trust between patients and staff. The stern approach is also at odds with the more empathetic treatment model Bernard has advocated as manager of the unit. He has developed a unique approach to acute inpatient psychiatric care that seeks to reduce restraints and violence on the unit through personalized de-escalation techniques. Rather than react harshly to every patient infraction by isolating or restraining them, Bernard instructs his staff to use communication to resolve disputes and discourage bad behavior. If patients become problematic, he assigns one, two, or even three mental health associates to shadow the patient throughout the day—reserving isolation and forced restraint as final recourse to dangerously violent behavior. Bernard's efforts have been very successful on Ward B and, as a result, he has been solicited by other hospitals in the area and around the country to give presentations on his approach. Nigerian American staff who do not share Bernard's cultural, educational, and class background do not see this as the proper way to deal with patients and argue that a strict approach will actually help patients more than what they view as a coddling approach.

Thus it appears that the complex cultural identities of the black African staff can complicate efforts by management and other clinical staff to create a more welcoming environment and improve patient-staff interaction. A common theme stressed by management on Ward B is the value that having racially and ethnically diverse staff can provide in furthering those ends. It is thought that having a certain degree of matching based on race, ethnicity, or cultural background can enhance trust and communication on the unit. However, the presence of staff that simultaneously occupy more than one identity dimension, such as the Nigerian Americans, makes the process of broadly matching on only one identity dimension, such as race, much more difficult.

For example, Meg, an American nurse on Ward B with predominantly Irish ancestry, often turns to one of the few black American mental health associates to accompany her when she goes to administer medication to black American patients.

> Where I'm a white nurse coming at, let's say it's a young black male that thinks that I don't have a clue what they're going through, I think I might tend to use some of the—I can't really say African American, we have a lot of African staff here, they're not African American—but I tend to use one of the black male staff as support sometimes. We all know each other very well, that sometimes I can use that person as a buffer zone. I'm just thinking in terms of administering medication, to have somebody come with me, so that if the person has paranoia and that paranoia is based around "You're just giving that to me because I'm black and you want to shut me down" that hopefully they might see that I'm with my co-worker who's also a black person like themselves. And that person can say "No, we only want to help you; calm down, you're making a big noise here." I'd say that having the cultural diversity on the unit is really helpful, just to have a backup like that.

Meg illustrates the specific value that racial and cultural matches can have in easing interactions between nurses and patients. Having a racially black mental health associate help her administer medication reduces any mistrust that might exist due to Meg's status as a white female psychiatric nurse. However, she is very sensitive to the possibility that black African staff might not be as effective in helping her build trust with black American patients. In her experience, the cultural differences between black Americans and black Africans are clearly evident and can hamper this process. She explains it this way: "All black people here are not even close to being all the same culture. That's something that I've learned from working here over the years, that there are people on both ends of the pole. Just because their skin color is the same has nothing to do with their cultural beliefs or behaviors."

The cultural distinctions between immigrant and American-born blacks at PPH closely follow the terrain mapped out by Waters (1999) and that observed at AMC1. West Indian staff I spoke with at PPH see black American staff and patients as having a weaker work ethic, a lower sense of personal responsibility, and a weaker emphasis on family values than West Indians like themselves. They also view black American patients as more likely to see racism and discrimination as an impediment to their economic mobility. African staff I spoke with view black American patients as lazy bearers of children out of wedlock.[15] On the unit, stereotypes like these create an environment in which black American patients can be openly hostile and distrustful of black African staff who they feel do not treat them fairly and where black African staff are less empathetic and helpful towards black American patients. As Meg notes, this conflict has at times even risen to a level of open hostility and anti-immigrant sentiment:

> If I ever hear somebody say "go back to Africa," it's an African American patient speaking to an African staff here that has an accent. There's also tension among, there are black Americans that will say to African staff here, "Why don't you go back to your country?" If there's any sort of racial tension in this hospital it's between the island people, the black Americans, and the Africans. There's some African staff that really look down on African Americans who are, you know, they talk about them having children out of wedlock and how people don't think that that's ok. And a good amount of the African staff that work here wouldn't live in [laugh] quote "black" areas.

This example of open hostility between immigrant and American blacks, though a rare occurrence on the unit, illustrates how cultural differences between groups of patients with shared racial identity can create tension and hostility. Any benefit that shared racial identity might provide can be rapidly sidelined when perceived cultural differences are large enough. This was the case on Ward B, where as Meg says, "the African staff seem to have more in common with the white American staff than they do with the black American staff. It's amazing!"

Fluidity: The Flexibility and Fluidity of Identity

Another situation that indicates the presence of hyperdiversity is when the connection between racial-ethnic identity and cultural characteristics breaks down due to the flexibility and fluidity of the patient's self-asserted racial-ethnic identity. Clinicians and support staff may have difficulty understanding whether a patient is a member of a particular group if they rely on their physical features or behavior rather than the patient's self-identification.

Racial and ethnic classification is a complicated, socially constructed process. Immigrants often identify with their local country, village, or tribe rather than ethnic or pan-ethnic identities (Bean and Tienda 1987; Sommers 1991; Espiritu 1992; Lopez and Espiritu 1997). As one of our clinician-informants jokingly said, "I always considered myself Peruvian; but when I moved to the United States for medical school I learned that I was actually 'Latino'!"

Because of interracial marriage and relations, the number of people with mixed heritage who have flexibility in how they identify racially is increasing (Zack 1992; Root 1992; Waters 1990). Moreover, racial categories themselves are historically contingent and without biological basis (Hochschild and Powell 2008; King 2000). The very existence of a given racial-ethnic category may be false or at least contested (Zack 2002; Hollinger 1995; Appiah 1996). Under these circumstances, the coherent existence of these groups is in question, and racial-ethnic group membership cannot be externally determined (ascribed).

These situations provided significant challenges to the clinicians in our study, who often face the difficult task of determining what role cultural factors play in the mental health and health care of their patients. These clinicians, who often have limited direct experience with patients of certain backgrounds, need to make decisions about diagnosis and treatment in short windows of time and with imperfect and, at times, contradictory information. Patients who don't fit neatly into a racial-ethnic-cultural box could be especially challenging.

For example, Dr. Jeffrey, a young white male (Jewish) psychiatry resident at a large academic hospital in Boston recently treated a young, biracial (black-white) woman who challenged his ability to deal with complex issues of identity. As he recounts,

> I have a patient right now who, her mother is white and her father is black, and she self-identifies as black. Growing up and in college, and in med school, I would always have about one black friend. I don't know how it would come out to about one. I would say that my personal experience with black people is quite personally minimal. In other words, I haven't had very many close friends who are black. So my cultural competency with African American, or blacks of wherever geographic location that

they're from, is a lot less than I would like. So trying to understand where my patient comes from, seeing as she self-identifies as black, but genetically, she, well, environmentally she's been raised in part by a Caucasian mother. So her identity, she will say, is kind of confused, and is not clear. I think that when I work with her, [I try] to not make any assumptions based on what she says. And she'll make kind of stereotypic comments. I'm trying to think [of] one that she said—"You can't really trust black guys," she says. And it's kind of hard to know what to do with that as a white clinician, as any clinician I guess.

Dr. Jeffrey's lack of personal experience with African Americans leads him to be extra careful and not make improper assumptions about how his patient's identity may bear on the case. This, combined with the complicated nature of her identity as a biracial woman who self-identifies as black, makes it difficult for him to understand the meaning of certain statements that may seem internally contradictory. As a result, he seems uncomfortable with "race talk" generally and moves to reject the rhetoric of coherent racial identities:

So, sitting with her and letting her talk and not making any statements, and trying to get to know her better as a black woman, or as a biracial—which is one of the worst terms. I don't know if you've met with Barbara [who is also biracial] yet, but we have a great time with *biracial*. It's like you can use the term *biracial,* and it could mean a million different things. But the way most people use it is black, white, put 'em together, you have biracial. But two cultures that are—and I don't know a way to say this—but bring them together, that's biracial. Yet we don't really think in those terms, and so we always laugh and have a good time with biracial people. And then, just using the word *black* also has a lot of weight to it. And it bothers me when people say African American for any black person, because I mean, there are millions of black people who are not from Africa and have no identification with Africa any longer. And, but, I don't know. I just hate terms, like I hate words to try to describe people where race—I'm not sure what a race is.

Instead of discussing the specifics of his patient's case, Dr. Jeffrey digresses into a discussion of his discomfort with the usage of racial labels. His reluctance to neatly label his patient's identity as biracial illustrates the contested and subjective nature of racial and ethnic identity.

Another example of how sensitive the process of applying racial labels can be in clinical settings occurred during my field work at PPH. During a three week stint on the unit, I met an eighteen-year-old black man named Jerome. Jerome was a big presence on the unit—a big kid, standing over six feet tall, with muscular arms and chest and corn-rowed braids. But his infectious smile, baby face, and repetitive fist-bumps every time he passed you by belied the fact that he had been hospitalized in psychiatric facilities off and on since he was fifteen years old, and at times over the past two weeks had needed up to two-on-one direct supervision on the unit to control his bouts of paranoia and frustration. I talked to him just about every day over the course of three weeks and saw him progress from nearly needing restraints during the first week, to performing freestyle raps, dancing, and playing John Madden Football on PlayStation3 the day before his discharge.

During this time, I became curious about Jerome's background: how long had he been sick, where were his family members, where did his family come from? In my conversations with him, I learned that he is from Dorchester and Mattapan, that he grew up in a very poor, violent neighborhood, and that his brother sells drugs.[16] When I asked him where he was from, he would just say here, or Boston, or Dorchester. He never gave me any indication that he was anything other than a multigenerational black American. He did not have an accent or a name that would suggest an immigrant background. I was curious about how black American patients interacted with immigrant patients and staff, so I asked around about Jerome's ethnic background. Everyone I spoke to told me they thought he was black American, and though some black patients can tend to have that street attitude, Jerome wasn't like that at all (even though he does love hip-hop and often talks with a little bit of street slang). Jalina, a twenty-four-year-old mixed-heritage (African, black American, and Mexican) mental health associate told me that she and some of the other female mental health associates did feel threatened by him because of his size and his unstable psychosis.

So it was much to my surprise that the day after he was discharged, I discovered through the survey instrument that a member of the study staff had him fill out the day before that he was not multigenerational American but of mixed Haitian and Honduran descent. Few if any people on the unit knew this or felt it was an important enough aspect of his biography or identity to reveal it to me in our conversations. That Jerome did not mention this to me either strongly suggests that it may not be an important aspect of his identity. His choice to speak of where he was from in very local terms is another strong indicator that he did not strongly identify with his immigrant background. But from the standpoint of racial and ethnic classification, it was clear that the staff on Ward B had a mistaken impression of Jerome's background. However, this technically mistaken impression was actually the correct one, because Jerome self-identified as a black American and did not emphasize his immigrant roots. Ultimately, the staff did not delve deeply into his racial and ethnic identity or make assumptions based on it—relying instead on his self-identification and actual behavior to guide them.

This example shows the importance of not relying on external racial and ethnic identity markers to generate assumptions about behavioral qualities and cultural orientations. On Ward B, these markers are relied on much less than personal interactions with patients and other salient cultural markers and group memberships. Because Ward B is an acute inpatient unit, clinic staff usually have five days to two weeks to interact with a patient, reducing the problems of time and efficiency pressures (although psychiatrists are still bound by these to a significant degree). Even though Jerome's surprising case did not have a negative impact on his treatment, it illustrates how complicated issues of culture and identity can be in environments of hyperdiversity.

Misapplication

Individuals, on average, may share a substantial core of cultural characteristics with other members of their group. But how can it be determined whether any given patient fits the pattern? Even if characteristics do roughly correspond to group membership and providers can accurately identify individual patients as group members, they must also be able to accurately determine which group members are likely to share the characteristics of the group.

Clinicians in our sample expressed difficulty in determining when it is appropriate to rely on that probability to make a medical or scientific decision about treatment and when to inquire more deeply to discover individual traits. This of course varies across disciplines. Psychologists and social workers who have long-term therapeutic relationships with their clients are in a much better position to take a more individual approach than psychiatrists and primary care providers whose time with each patient is more limited. This problem was highlighted by Dr. King, a white American female attending primary care physician at an outpatient clinic at a large academic hospital in Boston. When asked about cultural treatment guidelines for certain ethnic groups, she discussed dietary patterns as an example of a cultural trait that is often misapplied to individual patients: "Yes, I've seen it with diets. Well, a Latino diet is this, and we can look at the NIH pyramid for food, and this is the Latino pyramid, and this is—in some senses it's just a series of lined up stereotypes and nobody fits into any stereotype perfectly and you're not going to be competent in every culture."

Dr. King feels that having an ethnic food pyramid can stereotype individual patients whose diets differ from the norm of their group and that, ultimately, it is impractical to expect doctors to have cultural formulations available for every conceivable group they are likely to encounter. Instead, she favors a more individual approach that deals with these issues on a case by case basis:

> I think the best thing is to just have the patients guide you in each case because you can have a man or a woman who is a Latino and eats totally

different foods. So, stereotyping them, that they're going to eat these particular foods because they are Latino is not necessarily going to advance your cause any more. And again you are back to the basic problem: Who is the person and what is their sense of culture, whatever culture they are coming from? And that is the only thing that is really relevant—what framework they come from and what their personal background is—personal, cultural, genetic, and so on. Not so much whether they fit into a stereotyped culture that we think we might understand but they might be the exception to.

The patient in this case is correctly identified as a Hispanics/Latinos, but there is little way of knowing, without direct confirmation of the patient's actual diet, whether they fit the cultural pattern of Hispanics and Latinos in general. In these cases, Dr. King argues, more attention needs to be paid to the unique perspective that each individual brings to the clinical encounter. The patient may be the exception to the rule.

Another example of this dilemma was provided by Lynn, a white American third-year psychiatry resident in a large health-care network in Greater Boston. When asked about using an ethnic classification system to help make sense of her patient's cultural perspectives, she also argues that patients' individual experience is often more relevant than their group memberships:

I think that a classification system might be extremely difficult. I don't know how that would necessarily play out. Particularly, as you mentioned, if we just say "Asian," there's obviously huge diversity within that culture. Also individuals' experience, even in spite of an inclination to say that they belong to a group, their experience can be so much different than the experience of their peers within that group.

Similar to Dr. King, Lynn feels that within-group diversity makes the use of ethnic cultural classification systems ineffective. To illustrate the point, she offers the following example:

I have a patient right now—she's a married African American woman, Jehovah's Witness, and it's interesting because in medicine, I don't have to tell you this because you know it, there's a lot of, there can be a lot of conflict between the medical system and people who really ascribe to the Jehovah's Witness religion in terms of blood transfusion, etcetera. For her in particular, I'm treating her as a mental health provider and her family is very much against her taking medications and seeing a psychiatrist. So even though for her, as someone who practices, who is a Jehovah's Witness, even though she doesn't necessarily believe that taking medications or seeing a therapist, she doesn't think that that's a bad thing. Knowing that's a stress that her family puts on her, and knowing that she feels stigmatized by her family, it's helpful to be aware of that.

Lynn's patient does not fit the cultural norm commonly ascribed to Jehovah's Witnesses. Although she might say that she does not believe in medication and seeing a therapist, she doesn't think it's a bad thing and is willing to do it despite her faith and her family.

This example illustrates the multiple levels of cultural complexity present in many cases. If one were to apply a cultural classification scheme to this case, assumptions would be made based on either African American cultural cues or the cultural norms implied by the patient's religious background. In fact, neither her religious nor her ethnic identity provides much useful guidance. What this example shows is that contrary to what her religious or ethnic identity would imply, the patient defies convention by accepting the use of medication for her condition.

Conclusion

Cultural environments of hyperdiversity emerge in periods of rapid demographic change and challenge traditional understandings of race and ethnicity. The ecology of care in Boston (and in many large, diverse, segregated American cities) sorts patients into vastly different treatment settings, each with a distinctive, increasingly unstable, and evolving ethnoracial character.[17] For clinicians and support personnel in our study, efforts to understand the complex interactions among race, ethnicity, and culture are disrupted as distinctions based on phenotype or nationality are blurred and minimized. Instead, distinctions are made based on language, nationality, class status, illness category, and immigration status. These are more emergent forms of social categorization using broad language-based ethnic identities such as *Spanish-speaking patient,* broad class-based identities such as *free-care patient,*[18] or broad immigration based identities such as *Somali-Bantu refugee* to label patients and target care.

These emergent forms of social categorization are accompanied by resistance to using race and ethnicity as a basis for cultural assumptions. Clinicians and support staff we spoke with advocate an individualized approach to taking culture into account. They do not assert that culture does not matter, but instead argue that in their experience, broad, identity-based indicators of cultural difference are too blunt of an instrument; when used, the unique characteristics of individuals are lost. Although it is clear that ignoring group-based markers of cultural difference is also problematic, criteria need to be developed to distinguish between patients for whom conventional racial-ethnic-cultural categories make sense and those for whom they do not. More work needs to be done to determine when the use of group categorization for clinical purposes is appropriate.

The existence of cultural environments of hyperdiversity shows that efforts to improve cultural competency in health care should be sensitive to local variations in racial and ethnic boundary-making and relations. Common forms of group identities that are salient in one clinical context may not be in another. This is especially true in communities with great racial and ethnic diversity or in those experiencing rapid demographic change due to increased immigration or residential mobility.

Notes

1. White refers to non-Hispanic white.
2. In recent decades, ethnic differences between European groups became less prominent, and racial tensions between blacks and whites became more pronounced (see Waters 1990; Formisano 1991). Although Boston continues to have a very ethnically diverse population of European descent that tends to identify ethnically rather than racially, the violent disputes over busing in the 1970s and the continuing patterns of racial segregation present in the Boston metropolitan area show that a palpable black-white divide exists in the city.
3. The modern ethnic pentagon first appeared in the 1980 U.S. Census, ushered in by the Office of Management and Budget's Statistical Policy Directive No. 15, which specified that all federal agencies were to collect data under four racial and one ethnic headings. These stood until 1997, when Native Hawaiian–Pacific Islander became a fifth racial category and people were permitted to choose more than one race (Hattam 2005; for further critiques of these approaches, see Sundstrom 2002).
4. I named and developed the concept of hyperdiversity, independently, from my observations in the field and the analysis of data for this research project. The term *hyperdiversity* has been used by others in the social sciences in recent years, notably by the sociologist Michael Maly in his 2005 book *Beyond Segregation* and the geographer Ines Miyares in a 2005 article that uses the term to describe the neighborhood of Jackson Heights in Queens, New York. Neither of these authors elaborates on the meaning of the term or articulates its theoretical significance. Maly defines hyperdiverse as a neighborhood that is mixed on numerous demographic dimensions, yet shifting and complex.
5. As Jennifer Hochschild and Brenna Powell (2008) point out, the process of racial classification has been a shifting landscape throughout American history. Their analysis of U.S. Census racial categories from 1850 to 1930 shows that racial classifications have been much more unstable and inconsistent than is often recognized.
6. The legacy of racism and discrimination throughout American history forms the basis for the contemporary salience of modern racial and ethnic classification. Racial and ethnic classification should not be seen as purely a nominal exercise divorced from the material reality of race as a structural basis for social stratification and inequality (Sundstrom 2002; Smedley, Stith, and Nelson 2003).
7. The Office of Minority Health has instituted national standards on Culturally and Linguistically Appropriate Services (CLAS), which include involuntary mandates to provide culturally appropriate care or risk losing federal funds.

8. Scholars have addressed the conflation of race, ethnicity and culture in health care (Hunt and de Voogd 2005; Carpenter-Song et al. 2007; Kleinman and Benson 2006; Epstein 2007; Gravlee and Sweet 2008; Ong 1995) and in classification (Appiah 1996; Idler 2007; Sundstrom 2003; Root 2000; Zack 2002).

9. Cultural brokers are not always eager to perform this role (see also chapter 3, this volume). According to Dr. Desmond, some interpreters do not see this as their responsibility, while others eagerly volunteer cultural information during or after the clinical encounter.

10. Although Central American immigrants are a new and rapidly growing community in areas surrounding Neighborhood Health Center, significant numbers of Central American immigrants and refugees have lived in nearby cities such as Cambridge and Somerville since the 1980s.

11. This data is drawn from one of our field sites, an acute inpatient ward within a larger private psychiatric hospital located south of Boston. The question of whether trust is a major issue for black patients is an empirical question which I will bracket for the moment and elaborate on later.

12. Although it is true that some immigrants with dark skin have the potential to identify increasingly with black Americans (especially if they share residential space and similar class position), recent research has shown that they overwhelmingly reject racial categorization as black and instead maintain a strong identification with the pan-ethnic categories of Latino or Hispanic or with their home country (Roth 2006). Darker-skinned Puerto Rican and Dominican immigrants in particular can see their economic mobility impacted by their perceived race. Color does not affect their social networks and assimilation patterns (Roth 2006, iv).

13. Puerto Ricans outnumber Dominicans and all other Spanish-speaking patients, representing roughly 70 percent of the Spanish-speaking patient population. This is somewhat surprising considering that the hospital is located near a populous Dominican neighborhood. However, in interviews with numerous staff I was informed that most of the Spanish-speaking patients on the unit are brought from outside the immediate area, from places such as Lawrence and Springfield. In these areas outside Greater Boston, there is even less language capacity for the treatment of Spanish-speaking psychiatric patients. This leads emergency rooms and other institutions no choice but to send their patients closer to Boston for treatment, even if it makes family visits difficult and less frequent.

14. Recent research documents widespread stigma of individuals with mental illness and a lack of treatment infrastructure. There are .4 psychiatric beds per 10,000 population and only 100 working psychiatrists in the country, the most populous in Africa with 140 million residents (Eaton and Agomoh 2008). A recent large scale survey of Yoruba-speaking regions of Nigeria found that over 96 percent of respondents believe that people with mental illness are dangerous because of their violent behavior (Gureje et al. 2005)

15. I do not wish to generalize about the entire black American patient population at PPH. The example cited here refers explicitly to a subset of the black American patient population, namely young black American males (and females) who are characterized by staff on the unit alternatively as

street, aggressive, tough, or from the hood. These patients generally come from the largely minority inner city areas of Boston, and many have a very defensive, oppositional style of interacting with staff and other patients. Many have been homeless or have lived in group homes for long periods. Beyond issues of race, ethnicity, and culture, these patients are considered by staff to be generally distrusting of others on the unit. They often use the language of race to express that distrust.

16. It wasn't until I interviewed his nurse that I found out he was originally diagnosed with bipolar disorder and psychosis.

17. The demographics of our clinic sites are presented in another chapter.

18. Free Care is now known as Health Safety Net, but patients are commonly referred to by the old Free Care label.

References

Alba, Richard, and Nancy Denton. 2004. "Old and New Landscapes of Diversity: The Residential Patterns of Immigrant Minorities." In *Not Just Black and White: Historical and Contemporary Perspectives on Immigration, Race and Ethnicity in the United States*, edited by Nancy Foner and George Fredrickson. New York: Russell Sage Foundation.

Allen, James P., and Eugene Turner. 2004. "Boston's Emerging Ethnic Quilt: A Geographic Perspective." Unpublished manuscript. Presented at the Annual Meeting of the Population Association of America, Boston (April 1, 2004).

Appiah, Kwame Anthony. 1996. "Race, Culture, Identity: Misunderstood Connections." In *Color Conscious*, edited by Kwame Anthony Appiah and Amy Gutman. Princeton, N.J.: Princeton University Press.

———. 2006. *Cosmopolitanism: Ethics in a World of Strangers*. New York: W. W. Norton.

Bean, Frank, and Gillian Stevens. 2003. *America's Newcomers and the Dynamics of Diversity*. New York: Russell Sage Foundation.

Bean, Frank, and Marta Tienda. 1987. *Hispanic Population of the United States*. New York: Russell Sage Foundation.

Betancourt, Joseph R., Alexander R. Green, J. Emilio Carrillo, and Owusu Ananeh-Firempong II. 2003. "Defining Cultural Competence: A Practical Framework for Addressing Racial/Ethnic Disparities in Health and Health Care." *Public Health Reports (1974-)* 118(4): 293–302.

Bluestone, Barry, and Mary Huff Stevenson. 2000. *The Boston Renaissance: Race, Space, and Economic Change in an American Metropolis*. New York: Russell Sage Foundation.

Borovoy, Amy, and Janet Hine. 2008. "Managing the Unmanageable: Elderly Russian Jewish Emigrés and the Biomedical Culture of Diabetes Care." *Medical Anthropology Quarterly* 22(1): 1–26.

Brach, Cindy, and Irene Fraser. 2000. "Can Cultural Competency Reduce Racial and Ethnic Health Disparities? A Review and Conceptual Model." *Medical Care Research and Review* 57(1): 181–217.

Carpenter-Song, Elizabeth A., Megan Nordquest Schwallie, and Jeffrey Longhofer. 2007. "Cultural Competence Reexamined: Critique and Directions for the Future." *Psychiatric Services* 58(10): 1362–65.

Chang, Doris F., and Alexandra Berk. 2009. "Making Cross-Racial Therapy Work: A Phenomenological Study of Clients' Experiences of Cross-Racial Therapy." *Journal of Counseling Psychology* 56(4): 521–36.

Eaton, Julian, and Ahamefula Agomoh. 2008. "Developing Mental Health Services in Nigeria." *Social Psychiatry Psychiatric Epidemiology* 43(7): 552–58.

Epstein, Steven. 2007. *Inclusion: The Politics of Difference in Medical Research.* Chicago: University of Chicago Press.

Espiritu, Yen Le. 1992. *Asian American Panethnicity: Bridging Institutions and Identities.* Philadelphia: Temple University Press.

Flores, Glenn, Denise Gee, and Beth Kastner. 2000. "The Teaching of Cultural Issues in U.S. and Canadian Medical Schools." *Academic Medicine* 75(5): 451–55.

Foner, Nancy, and George Fredrickson, eds. 2004. *Not Just Black and White: Historical and Contemporary Perspectives on Immigration, Race, and Ethnicity in the United States.* New York: Russell Sage Foundation.

Ford, Julian D. 2008. "Trauma, Posttraumatic Stress Disorder, and Ethnoracial Minorities: Toward Diversity and Cultural Competence in Principles and Practices." *Clinical Psychology: Science and Practice* 15(1): 35–61.

Formisano, Ronald. 1991. *Boston Against Busing: Race, Class, and Ethnicity in the 1960's and 1970's.* Chapel Hill: University of North Carolina Press.

Fox, Kenneth. 1995. "Anthropology's Hoodoo Museum." *Culture, Medicine and Psychiatry* 19(3): 409–21.

Geertz, Clifford. 1960. "The Javanese Kijaji: The Changing Role of a Cultural Broker." *Comparative Studies in Society and History* 2(2): 228–49.

Good, Byron J. 1977. "The Heart of What's the Matter: Semantics and Illness in Iran." *Culture, Medicine and Psychiatry* 1(1): 25–58.

———. 1994. *Medicine, Rationality, and Experience.* New York: Cambridge University Press.

Good, Byron J., and Mary-Jo DelVecchio Good. 1980. "The Meaning of Symptoms: A Cultural Hermeneutic Model for Clinical Practice." In *The Relevance of Social Science for Medicine,* edited by Leon Eisenberg and Arthur Kleinman. Dordrecht, Neth.: D. Reidel.

———. 1981. "The Semantics of Medical Discourse." In *Sciences and Cultures. Sociology of the Sciences,* vol. 5, edited by Everett Mendelsohn and Yehúda Elkana. Dordrecht, Neth.: D. Reidel.

Good, Mary-Jo DelVecchio, Cara James, Byron J. Good, and Anne E. Becker. 2003. "The Culture of Medicine and Racial, Ethnic, and Class Disparities in Healthcare." In *Unequal Treatment: Confronting Racial and Ethnic Disparities in Health Care,* edited by Brian D. Smedley, Adrienne Y. Stith, and Alan Ray Nelson. Washington, D.C.: National Academies Press.

Gravlee, Clarence C., and Elizabeth Sweet. 2008. "Race, Ethnicity, and Racism in Medical Anthropology, 1977–2002." *Medical Anthropology Quarterly.* 22(1): 27–51.

Guarnaccia, Peter, and Orlando Rodriguez. 1996. "Concepts of Culture and their Role in the Development of Culturally-Competent Mental Health Services." *Hispanic Journal of Behavioral Sciences* 18(4): 419–43.

Guarnaccia, Peter, William Vega, and Robert Bonner. 2006. "Improving Quality of Care Through Cultural Competence: Building a Long-Range Strategy for Organizational Change." Unpublished manuscript.

Gureje, Oye, Victor O. Lasebikan, Olusola Ephraim-Oluwanuga, Benjamin O. Olley, and Lola Kola. 2005. "Community Study of Knowledge of and Attitude to Mental Illness in Nigeria." *British Journal of Psychiatry* 2005(5): 436–41.

Hattam, Victoria. 2005. "Ethnicity and the Bounds of Race: Reading Directive 15." *Daedalus* 134(1): 61–69.

Hochschild, Jennifer L., and Brenna M. Powell. 2008. "Racial Reorganization and the United States Census 1850–1930: Mulattoes, Half-Breeds, Mixed Parentage, Hindoos, and the Mexican Race." *Studies in American Political Development* 22(1): 59–96.

Hollinger, David. 1995. *Postethnic America.* New York: Basic Books.

Hunt, Linda M. 2005. "Health Research: What's Culture Got to Do with It?" *Lancet* 366(9486): 617–18.

Hunt, Linda M., and Katherine B. de Voogd. 2005. "Clinical Myths of the Cultural 'Other': Implications for Latino Patient Care." *Academic Medicine* 80(10): 617–18.

Idler, Jose Enrique. 2007. *Officially Hispanic.* Lanham, Md.: Lexington Books.

Kagawa-Singer, Marjorie, and Shaheen Kassim-Lakha. 2003. "A Strategy to Reduce Cross-Cultural Miscommunication and Increase the Likelihood of Improving Health Outcomes." *Academic Medicine* 78(6): 577–87.

Kim, Bryan S. K., Peggy H. Yang, Donald R. Atkinson, Maren M. Wolfe, and Sehee Hong. 2001. "Cultural Value Similarities and Differences Among Asian American Ethnic Groups." *Cultural Diversity and Ethnic Minority Psychology* 7(4): 343–61.

King, Desmond S. 2000. *Making Americans: Immigration, Race, and the Origins of the Diverse Democracy.* Cambridge, Mass.: Harvard University Press.

Kirmayer, Laurence, and Norman Sartorius. 2007. "Cultural Models and Somatic Syndromes." *Psychosomatic Medicine* 69(9): 832–40.

Kleinman, Arthur. 1980. *Patients and Healers in the Context of Culture.* Berkeley: University of California Press.

Kleinman, Arthur, and Peter Benson. 2006. "Anthropology in the Clinic: The Problem of Cultural Competency and How to Fix It." *PLoS medicine* 3: e294. Available at: http://www.plosmedicine.org/article/info%3Adoi%2F10.1371%2Fjournal.pmed.0030294 (accessed March 21, 2009).

Kleinman, Arthur, Leon Eisenberg, and Byron J. Good. 1978. "Culture, Illness, and Care: Clinical Lessons from Anthropological and Cross-Cultural Research." *Annals of Internal Medicine* 88(2): 251–58.

Lakes, Kimberly, Steven Lopez, and Linda C. Garro. 2006. "Cultural Competence and Psychotherapy: Applying Anthropologically Informed Conceptions of Culture." *Psychotherapy: Theory Research, Practice, Training* 43(4): 380–96.

Lambo, Thomas A. 1956. "Neuropsychiatric Observations in the Western Region of Nigeria." *British Medical Journal* 2(5006): 1388–394.

Lo, Ming-Cheng Miriam. 2010. "Cultural Brokerage: Creating Linkages Between Voices of Lifeworld and Medicine in Cross-Cultural Clinical Settings." *Health:* 14(5): 484–504.

Lo, Ming-Cheng M., and Clare Stacey. 2008. "Beyond Cultural Competency: Bourdieu, Patients and Clinical Encounters." *Sociology of Health & Illness* 30(5): 741–55.

Logan, John, Deirdre Oakley, and Jacob Stowell. 2003. "Segregation in Neighborhoods and Schools: Impacts on Minority Children in the Boston

Region." Paper presented at the "Color Lines" Conference, sponsored by the Civil Rights Project, Harvard University (August 30–September 1). Produced by the Lewis Mumford Center for Comparative Urban and Regional Research.

Lopez, David, and Yen Le Espiritu. 1997. "Panethnicity in the United States." In *New American Destinies,* edited by Darrell Hamamoto and Rodolfo Torres. New York: Routledge.

Maly, Michael T. 2005. *Beyond Segregation: Multiracial and Multiethnic Neighborhoods in the United States.* Philadelphia: Temple University Press.

Maramba, Gloria Gia, and Gordon C. Nagayama Hall. 2002. "Meta-Analyses of Ethnic Match as a Predictor of Dropout, Utilization, and Level of Functioning." *Cultural Diversity and Ethnic Minority Psychology* 8(3): 290–97.

Massey, Douglas, ed. 2008. *New Faces in New Places.* New York: Russell Sage Foundation.

Metzl, Jonathan M. 2010. *The Protest Psychosis—How Schizophrenia Became a Black Disease.* Boston: Beacon Press.

Miyares, Ines. 2005. "From Exclusionary Covenant to Ethnic Hyperdiversity in Jackson Heights, Queens." *Geographical Review* 94(4): 462–83.

Ng, Bernardo, Joel Dimsdale, G. Paul Shragg, Reena Deutsch. 1996. "Ethnic Differences in Analgesic Consumption for Postoperative Pain." *Psychosomatic Medicine* 58(2): 125–29.

Nichter, Mark. 1981. "Idioms of Distress: Alternatives in the Expression of Psychosocial Distress: A Case Study from South India." *Culture, Medicine & Psychiatry* 5(4): 379–408.

Nobles, Melissa. 2000. *Shades of Citizenship: Race and the Census in Modern Politics.* Palo Alto, Calif.: Stanford University Press.

Ong, Aihwa. 1995. "Making the Biopolitical Subject: Cambodian Immigrants, Refugee Medicine, and Cultural Citizenship in California." *Social Science & Medicine* 40(9): 1243–57.

Pole, Nnamdi, Joe P. Gone, and Madhur Kulkarni. 2008. "Posttraumatic Stress Disorder Among Ethnoracial Minorities in the United States." *Clinical Psychology: Science and Practice* 15(1): 35–61.

Prewitt, Kenneth. 2005. "Racial Classification in America: Where Do We Go from Here?" *Daedalus* 134(1): 5–17.

———. 2009. "Does (Should) Racial Counting Have a Future in America?" Lecture presented at the John F. Kennedy School of Government, Harvard University. Cambridge, Mass. (February 23).

Root, Maria. 1992. *Racially Mixed People in America.* Newbury Park, Calif.: Sage Publications.

Root, Michael. 2000. "How We Divide the World." *Philosophy and Science* 67(suppl): S28–S639.

Roth, Wendy. 2006. "Caribbean Race and American Dreams: How Migration Shapes Dominicans' and Puerto Ricans' Racial Identities and its Impact on Socioeconomic Mobility." Ph.D. dissertation, Harvard University.

Santiago-Irizarry, Vilma. 2001. *Medicalizing Ethnicity: The Construction of Latino Identity in a Psychiatric Setting.* Ithaca, N.Y.: Cornell University Press.

Shaw, Susan. 2005. "The Politics of Recognition in Culturally Appropriate Care." *Medical Anthropology Quarterly* 19(3): 290–309.

Shea, Jennifer, and Charles Jones. 2006. "Latinos in Massachusetts: A Mid-Decade Status Report." A report for the Mauricio Gaston Institute.

Shin, Sung-Man, Clifton Chow, Teresita Camacho-Gonsalves, Rachel J. Levy, Elaine I. Allen, and Stephen H. Leff. 2005. "A Meta-Analytic Review of Racial-Ethnic Matching for African American and Caucasian American Clients and Clinicians." *Journal of Counseling Psychology* 52(1): 45–56.

Smedley, Brian D., Adrienne Y. Stith, and Alan Ray Nelson. 2003. *Unequal Treatment: Confronting Racial and Ethnic Disparities in Health Care.* Washington, D.C.: National Academies Press.

Sommers, Laurie Kay. 1991. "Inventing Latinismo: The Creation of 'Hispanic' Panethnicity in the United States." *Journal of American Folklore* 104(411): 32–53.

Sue, Stanley. 1998. "In Search of Cultural Competence in Psychotherapy and Counseling." *American Psychologist* 53(4): 440–48.

Sundstrom, Ronald. 2002. "Racial Nominalism." *Journal of Social Philosophy* 33(2): 193–210.

———. 2003. "Race and Place: Social Space in the Production of Human Kinds." *Philosophy & Geography* 6(1): 83–95.

Taylor, Janelle S. 2003. "The Story Catches You and You Fall Down: Tragedy, Ethnography, and 'Cultural Competence.'" *Medical Anthropology Quarterly* 17(2): 159–81.

Vega, William. 2005. "Higher Stakes for Cultural Competence." *General Hospital Psychiatry* 27(6): 446–50.

Waters, Mary C. 1990. *Ethnic Options: Choosing Identities in America.* Berkeley: University of California Press.

———. 1999. *Black Identities: West Indian Immigrant Dreams and American Realities.* Cambridge, Mass.: Harvard University Press.

———. 2008. "Counting and Classifying by Race: The American Debate." *The Tocqueville Review* 29(1): 1–21.

Waters, Mary, Reed Ueda, and Helen Marrow, eds. 2007. *The New Americans: A Guide to Immigration Since 1965.* Cambridge, Mass.: Harvard University Press

Wilson, William Julius, and Richard Taub. 2006. *There Goes the Neighborhood: Racial, Ethnic, and Class Tensions in Four Chicago Neighborhoods.* New York: Alfred A. Knopf.

Winant, Howard. 2000. "Race and Race Theory." *Annual Review of Sociology* 26: 169–85.

Zack, Naomi. 1992. *Race and Mixed Race.* Philadelphia: Temple University Press.

———. 2002. *Philosophy of Race and Science.* New York: Routledge.

Chapter 3

Pas de Trois: Medical Interpreters, Clinical Dilemmas, and the Patient-Provider-Interpreter Triad

SARAH S. WILLEN

> The whole relationship with the interpreter, both for the patient and the provider, is predicated on trust; you trust the interpreter is going to be skilled, that they're going to be accurate, that they're not going to bring into it their own biases and interject their own opinions. . . . [E]verybody has to give up a little bit in order for it to really work.
> —Manager of interpreter services at a New England hospital

A S MORE and more patients with limited English proficiency (LEP) arrive at United States health centers seeking medical care, many patient-provider dyads are expanding to include an additional party—a medical interpreter. For all parties involved, this substantive change in the traditional provider-patient dyad involves an array of new and distinct clinical challenges. This chapter considers the dynamics and complexities of this emerging clinical pas de trois (Wadensjö 1998).

This chapter draws on thirteen interviews conducted with professional medical interpreters employed at four health-care settings, including two academic medical centers, a community health center with a generic orientation, and a community health center that places particular emphasis on culturally sensitive care.[1] For these institutions, offering interpreter services constitutes a clear and direct effort to respond proactively to the complicated clinical and practical implications of the growing hyperdiversity within their patient populations. Interviewees include interpreters born in the United States (including Puerto Rico) and others born overseas—in Guatemala, Cape Verde, Haiti, Lebanon, and Japan. Some are native speakers of the languages for which they interpret; others were raised in bilingual households; and still others are native English speakers who acquired a second language while studying or working abroad. Languages represented include Spanish (eight interpreters), Portuguese (Brazilian and Portuguese dialects) (two), Cape Verdean (a Portuguese creole) (one), Haitian Kreyol (one), Arabic (one), Japanese (one), and American Sign Language (one).[2] A number of foreign-born interviewees trained as physicians in their countries of origin and now work as medical interpreters while preparing for recertification in the United States. Others have no formal medical background but came to the interpreting profession from other fields; one had worked as a court interpreter, another as a Peace Corps volunteer, and a third was a college student with plans to attend medical school. Several had taken professional interpretation courses at local colleges or medical centers, and one had a university degree in medical interpretation. Other interpreters—especially those who joined the profession before the mid-2000s—possessed little or no formal training, only the requisite language skills. Three interviewees served as administrative directors of the interpreter service units at their respective health care institutions.

The Growing Role of the Medical Interpreter

Medical interpreters, who play a relatively new role in the U.S. health-care system, are fast becoming key members of clinical care teams. One reason for the growth of the medical interpreter role is the rapid and recent demographic change associated with growing hyperdiversity within the United States. Whereas 4.8 percent of the population spoke English "less than very well" in 1980, that number had risen to 6.1 percent by 1990 and to 8.1 percent—approximately 21 million people—by 2000 (Shin and Bruno 2003). The demand for interpreter services is especially high in areas with substantial immigrant populations, such as Massachusetts, where individuals with low English proficiency amount to 8.6 percent of the population (U.S. Census Bureau 2010).[3]

Another factor contributing to the growth of this new clinical role is the growing recognition that alternatives to professional interpretation involve myriad practical, technical, and ethical problems. Many health-care institutions across the United States still lack formal interpreter services and, as a result, are left with little choice but to call on "dual role interpreters" (Moreno, Otero-Sabogal, and Newman 2007) such as hospital staff members—including administrative or housekeeping staff with little or no medical knowledge—or patients' relatives (including children in many cases). As Maria Moreno and her colleagues point out, "interpretation is a learned skill; whereas it is true that every interpreter can speak at least two languages, it does not follow that every bilingual person is an effective interpreter" (2007, 331). Ad hoc interpreters are prone to omitting, adding, substituting, and volunteering information (Dye 2001; Fernandez et al. 2004; Flores et al. 2003; Haffner 1992; Hampers and McNulty 2002; Timmins 2002; Woloshin et al. 1997), and, in many cases, untrained interpreters "succumb to the temptation to . . . informally mediate, rather than interpret, information" (Moreno, Otero-Sabogal, and Newman 2007, 331; see also Sampson 2006). Reliance on family members, and especially children, has been identified as particularly problematic (National Health Law Program and The Access Project 2003; Office of Minority Health 2001).

Third, professional interpreters' organizations have succeeded in convincing many health care institutions and policymakers of the importance of their services—in part by emphasizing the problems associated with ad hoc alternatives. These efforts have benefited, in particular, from a fourth factor: a wave of increased government interest in, and attention to, the need for interpreter services. Justification for requiring interpreter services can be traced to the 1964 Civil Rights Act (Title VI section 601), which prohibits discrimination in the distribution of federally funded services. More specific federal regulations concerning provision of interpreter services were developed under President Bill Clinton (see Executive Order 13166) and under the Department of Health and Human Services guidelines (Section VI.A, dated August 30, 2000) (Moreno, Otero-Sabogal, and Newman 2007). Formal policies vary considerably by state, with especially strong commitments to the provision of interpreter services on the books in California, Minnesota, Pennsylvania, and Massachusetts (Chen, Youdelman, and Brooks 2007; Mayer and Villaire 2007, 256; Perkins and Youdelman 2006). In Massachusetts, for instance, medical interpreters and other advocacy groups were successful in lobbying for legislation that, since 2001, has required the provision of competent medical interpreters—defined as interpreters who possess fluency in both English and the target language as well as familiarity with medical terms—in both emergency and acute psychiatric settings.

Despite this proliferation of state and federal laws, "current policies are limited and unclear as to what constitutes appropriate language services" (Moreno, Otero-Sabogal, and Newman 2007, 331). As the National Health Law Program has pointed out, numerous federal and state laws have been enacted to protect LEP speakers from health-related discrimination (Perkins, Youdelman, and Wong 2003; see also ACORN 2004). Yet these legal statues and obligations are still unfamiliar to many

clinicians and health care organizations—not to mention many patie
(Chen, Youdelman, and Brooks 2007).

Medical Interpretation:
A Growing Literature

A growing body of clinical, legal, and sociolinguistic research supports
the inclusion of professional interpreters in clinical settings and simultaneously highlights the practical challenges and dilemmas associated with
their presence. In the clinical domain, research suggests that reliance on
ad hoc interpreters (as opposed to professional interpreters) can lead to
an increase in clinically consequential errors (Flores et al. 2003; National
Health Law Program and National Council on Interpreting in Health
Care 2007) and otherwise impair clinical care (Baker, Hayes, and Fortier
1998; Kaplan, Greenfield, and Ware. 1989; Takka 1991; Woloshin et al.
1995). Some evidence indicates that reliance on trained interpreters can
lead to significantly higher utilization rates for preventive services and
follow-up care (Jacobs et al. 2001).

Within the field of health law, legal scholars and clinicians have produced systematic reviews of the state and federal statutes requiring the
provision of interpreter services and analyzed policy initiatives designed
to achieve substantive improvement in health care for LEP patients
(Chen et al. 2007; National Health Law Program and National Council on
Interpreting in Health Care 2007; National Health Law Program and The
Access Project 2003; Perkins and Youdelman 2006; Perkins, Youdelman,
and Wong 2003). Although interpreters may once have constituted a bou-
tique service at American hospitals and clinics, growing hyperdiversity
means that the interpreter role is growing in importance. Moreover, the
stakes of finding successful models for integrating interpreters into clinical encounters are on the rise.

Sociolinguists and interpretation studies scholars have analyzed specific challenges associated with the interpretation process and debated
how active and visible a role interpreters ought to play in interpreted
interactions (Angelelli 2004a, 2004b; Bot 2005; Davidson 2000; Kaufert
and Putsch 1997; Wadensjö 1998). For instance, interpreters sometimes
answer, instead of asking, questions; offer incomplete translations, especially when clinicians ask multipart questions; or translate incorrectly,
sometimes as a result of the technical nature of clinician's questions
or patients' limited language proficiency (Prince 1986, cited in Angelelli
2004a). Overall, however, relatively few studies have explored either the
actual practice of clinical interpretation or the impact of this triadic relationship on care (Jacobs et al. 2006). Exceptions include several studies
in mental health settings (Drennan and Swartz 2002; Miller et al. 2007;
Tribe and Rayal 2002).

Health-care providers have responded in different ways to the increasing presence of interpreters within clinical settings. Although this chapter focuses on interpreter perspectives, it is helpful to reflect momentarily on the clinician perspectives that emerged in the study (see also chapter 6, this volume). Some of the clinicians interviewed suggested that the presence of a medical interpreter disrupts the clinical power dynamic, in which the clinician is supposed to be the expert. One expressed frustration at feeling at "the mercy of the interpreters." Others, however, welcomed this new dynamic and the opportunities it can present for learning about cultural differences and refining their communication techniques.

Models of Interpretation: Conduit? Detective? Robot? Ghost?

Despite the growing need for skilled medical interpreters, and despite the growing number of training programs and professional organizations for interpreters, most aspects of the profession currently are not standardized in the United States (Moreno, Otero-Sabogal, and Newman 2007). No standardized curriculum for interpreter training and education, no universally recognized diploma or certification, and—perhaps most significantly—no single model that defines and delimits the interpreter role exists. As a result, individual interpreters tend to understand and enact their professional roles in substantially different ways. Not only do models of interpretation vary but, as elaborated upon in the following section, models also vary in accordance with health-care centers' distinct institutional cultures.

Multiple metaphors have been used to characterize the ideal role of the medical interpreter in clinical interactions (Angelelli 2004a, 129–32, 2004b, 19–20; Roy 2002). Such metaphors hint at the multiplicity of interpretive models currently in play. These metaphors can be organized in several clusters: mechanical metaphors (machine, telephone, modem, robot), metaphors of connection and facilitation (channel, conduit, bridge, clarifier), and metaphors of exploration and investigation (detective, mine digger, diamond connoisseur). Rather than representing discrete or distinct models, these metaphors instead highlight core dilemmas that interpreters grapple with and shed light on key issues that divide the profession into different schools of thought.

Mechanical Metaphors

Mechanical metaphors presume that interpreters play a strictly technical role. They rest on an assumption that linguistic content should be translated literally, and that interpreters can isolate the meaning of a statement without concern that multiple interpretations are possible. As a result, models grounded in these metaphors may remain faithful to an ideology of linguistic precision, but they tend to neglect two key issues: first, that interpreters inevitably make interpretive choices, and, second, that these choice-making processes inevitably render interpreters co-participants in the production of clinic-based discourse (Angelelli 2004b, 14). Another common feature of machine-based models is an insistence upon maximum interpreter invisibility. This demand for invisibility emerges most clearly in discussions of interpreter as "ghost" (Kopczynski 1994, 192–95, cited in Alexieva 2002). Angelelli calls this the "myth of invisibility" and argues that it has a variety of effects, some positive and some negative—and some of which may be advantageous under certain circumstances and disadvantageous in others. For instance, the myth of invisibility promotes an image of interpreters as neutral rather than aligned with the clinical team; its aim is to neutralize their social power within clinical interactions. At the same time, by absolving interpreters of responsibility for the outcome of such interactions, it can, at least theoretically, lower the stakes of their engagement and their level of investment. Although the push for invisibility is meant to foreground patients' and clinicians' voices by preventing interpreters from imposing their own views on the clinical encounter, it can impair the flow of information and the cultivation of clinical rapport. Additionally, this emphasis on invisibility is not exclusive to mechanical models; it is also linked to some metaphors of connection and facilitation—especially those that identify the interpreter as a "conduit" or "channel."

Despite the epistemological, practical, and ethical problems it can generate, the professional model of interpreter as a kind of invisible machine, conduit, or ghostly presence is written into many professional associations' standards of practice—including those of the Massachusetts Medical Interpreting Association (MMIA) and the California Health Care Interpreters Association (CHIA), among others—as well as many interpreter training courses (Angelelli 2004b, 20–22). Students may be told, for instance, "Your job is to grasp the meaning and state it in the other language. You have no part in what is said" (21). As Angelelli notes, "by stating that the interpreter's responsibility is to convey the *meaning of the message* into another language we are denying the fact that meaning is not monolithic and that all parties to a conversation work together . . . to generate this meaning" (2004b, 20; emphasis in original).

Metaphors of Connection and Facilitation

Other models are more attentive to the co-constructive dimensions of the interpreter role. Models that draw on the second set of metaphors—of interpreter as facilitator or bridge—emphasize the need to understand not only the linguistic content, but also the cultural context of a speaker's words. According to these models, interpreters are expected to help care-seeking patients and knowledgeable providers connect not just linguistically, but also conceptually. To maximize mutual comprehensibility, they are expected to translate not only words, but also ideas, concepts, and therapeutic goals across cultural worldviews. These worldviews include the personal cultural background of patient and provider and the culture of medicine, as well as the culture of the layperson.

Models based on connection and facilitation are notable for their attention to the importance of sociolinguistic context and their recognition that literal translation of linguistic content can leave critical questions unanswered and lead to misunderstandings when no equivalent concepts exist across languages, or when an interpreter feels disempowered and unable to request clarification. At the same time, however, such models can also put interpreters in positions of undue—or undesired—responsibility, and they involve a risk, at least in theory, of allowing the interpreter's voice to overwhelm that of either the clinician or the patient.

Metaphors of Exploration and Investigation

A third constellation of metaphors—those involving exploration and investigation (for example, detective, mine digger, and diamond connoisseur)—suggests an even more active role for interpreters. From this perspective, responsibilities such as digging, sifting, or sorting through spoken language are part and parcel of the interpretive role. Models based on these metaphors may or may not involve explicit recognition of the co-constructive dimensions of interpretation noted above. As suggested, active pursuit of clinically relevant information may run the risk of compromising an interpreter's neutrality by aligning him or her more strongly with one of the two core parties in the clinical interaction. Also, although clinical discourse is not supposed to take on adversarial tones, it occasionally does (Kaufert and Putsch 1997). Under such circumstances, shifts in social footing that strengthen the clinician's role—including a patient's perception that the ostensibly neutral third party in the room (the interpreter) is aligned with the clinician—can generate the unintended consequences of silencing or otherwise disempowering the patient.

This cluster of metaphors grants interpreters license to probe actively for information that clinicians or patients may have overlooked and, moreover, to contribute to the clinical interaction by volunteering information deemed relevant for contextual or clarifying purposes. Active exploration and investigation of this sort can prove beneficial when other differences between clinicians and providers, for instance, in terms of educational level, scientific literacy, and cultural background, might impede comprehension, diagnosis, treatment, or clinician-patient rapport.

Unlike mechanical approaches, models of this sort do involve the risk that interpreters' perspectives might overwhelm the voice of either the clinician or the patient.

Interpreter As Advocate

An important final model merits mention as well: the potential for interpreters to serve explicitly as advocates. Interpreters—and researchers—hold varied opinions concerning the relationship between medical interpretation and patient advocacy. Those who advocate strict adherence to models of interpreter invisibility tend to oppose active advocacy efforts, whereas those who view interpreters as co-participants in clinical discourse and co-constructors of meaning are more likely to support them.

Advocacy can carry a wide variety of meanings and imply a wide variety of activities either on behalf of individual patients (and possibly their families) or, alternatively, on behalf of cultural or linguistic communities for whom language barriers impede access to health care services. For example, patient advocacy might involve speaking up when a patient appears not to have understood an explanation or set of instructions, protesting (perhaps subtly) when a doctor acts in a patronizing manner toward a patient, helping a patient navigate the health-care bureaucracy, making phone calls or writing letters on a patient's behalf, accompanying the patient to other appointments within or beyond the walls of the health-care institution, or engaging in community-level consciousness-raising campaigns about the availability of health-care services. In some forms, this model of interpretation may map onto the role of culture broker.

Mixing and Matching of Models

The prevailing lack of consensus concerning the ideal interpreter role helps explain why models become mixed-and-matched both in training programs for professional interpreters and in the realm of everyday interpretive practice. One interpreter interviewed for this study, who interprets in Spanish and Portuguese at a large academic medical center, offered an especially clear illustration of this mix-and-match approach. His characterization of the interpreter role, still crisp in his mind from the training course he had taken, involved four basic elements:

> Well, the basics of being an interpreter—there are four roles: you're supposed to be a *conduit* of information, you're supposed to be a *clarifier*, you're supposed to be a *cultural broker*, and lastly, but most importantly I think, you're supposed to be an *advocate*. So those are the four things that they really kind of instilled in us. (emphasis added)

For this interpreter, these functions are not isolated or separate from one another; rather they constitute complementary dimensions of a single professional role. "I think that they're all combined into one," he continued,

> because I feel that when I explain something . . . to the patient I am being a conduit of information, I am conveying actually what the doctor wanted me to say to the patient. I am being a clarifier for sure. I am being a cultural broker—not necessarily in terms of like, American versus Columbian culture, but between like biomedical culture versus people who don't know anything about medicine.

This expansive understanding of the interpreter role, however, is not universally shared. Another interviewee, an American Sign Language (ASL) interpreter at another academic medical center, described an instance in which considerable differences of opinion arose. He had recently attended a conference for interpreters at which different philosophies of interpreting were discussed and debated.

> Last year there was a really, almost like this fallout. This one guy . . . was saying that interpreters should be robots basically, that we should just, we should not think about patient safety or anything about culture. We should just say exactly, we should represent exactly what people say . . . but most people don't agree with that, you know? Most people realize you should think about the safety, the safety of the person.

When asked whether he thought it was appropriate for interpreters to take on a patient advocacy role, he explained, "I think you should always think of safety, definitely that has to be the big thing, you know . . . You don't want to break confidentiality but you should try to be safe." He went on to describe a case in which a deaf patient had seen a physician without an interpreter and the physician had prescribed a blood thinner without knowing that the patient was already taking one. Soon thereafter, an interpreter bumped into the patient in the hall, learned of the new prescription, and took the patient back to the physician to clarify. With the interpreter's intervention, the physician realized his error and said, "Oh, I realize it's not a good idea to do these appointments without an interpreter." For our interviewee, the interpreter in question had definitely done the right thing by asking questions and taking on an advocacy role: "If he had just said oh well . . . this person is not on my schedule so I'm just going to leave, . . . the patient, he could've ended up dying." This added concern—that literal or robotic interpretation might place patients in clinical, even mortal danger—highlights yet another problem with the invisibility model that merits greater attention in future research.

As these brief comments suggest, the role of the medical interpreter, although growing in prominence and professionalization, is still very much up for grabs. Furthermore, as discussed in the next section, the health-care institutions that served as sites for our study tend to promote substantially different models of the interpreter role.

Divergent Interpretation Models

Some of the most salient differences among health-care institutions emerged during the interviews our study team conducted with three administrative managers of interpreter service units. Two were employed at academic medical centers, and one worked at a community clinic in an ethnically hyperdiverse area of Boston. Each manager spoke explicitly about the differences among the various institutions' ideal models for the interpreter role.

Academic Medical Center 1: A Low-Advocacy, Black Box Model

The manager at one of the academic medical centers contrasted two basic approaches: her hospital's approach, on one hand, and the approach employed by community health centers and a local community-oriented teaching hospital, on the other. Although the interpreter services unit she manages tends toward the invisible conduit end of the spectrum, these other institutions

> do believe in advocacy. Their interpreters are patient advocates. And we differ in that model, a little bit. . . . You will see more of the advocates and outreach workers in the health centers. This is how they kind of like 'get' the position, how people are . . . starting to fulfill all these needs. But for the most part, the other hospitals only have interpreters, not something else.

She attributed this difference, at least in part, to the exponentially higher volume of patients at her institution versus smaller community health centers. Beyond this technical consideration, however, she also expressed principled opposition to more advocacy-oriented models:

> Some of the things I believe the community health centers are doing is, they have more involvement, I believe, in the care of the patient. That might or might not work. Because . . . you're making the [patient] become very dependent on you, instead of trying to teach them how to be independent. So they're doing everything for them . . . what they call patient navigators . . . take them and bring them to all their appointments instead of like, "Okay, let's do it once, let me show you how to do this, and then you're on your own." And that's how you become independent. I believe they do take the patients under their wing. But again, also by the nature of their business, it's really small. . . . They might have, what, I don't know, . . . about five to six thousand cases per year, when we see a hundred thousand.

In other words, this manager felt that patients should not rely too heavily on interpreters; instead, interpreters should actively promote patient independence for both practical and moral reasons.

Academic Medical Center 2: "We're In the Middle"

The director of interpreter services at a second academic medical center, in contrast, explained that her institution fits in between two extremes. "I always say that we're in the middle," she said.

> So my dear colleague at [the other hospital] is a proponent of sort of the black box model. So, "do not sit with the patient in the waiting room, and do not converse because then you put yourself, the interpreter, in danger of hearing something that the patient may not want you to convey and then you're sort of in trouble."

To illustrate her point, she described a situation in which a patient might tell an interpreter something she wants to conceal from her clinician.

> So let's say you're in the waiting room and the patient says—which has happened to interpreters—"You know my son-in-law's hitting me at home. Don't tell. It'll get worse. I just told you. If I wanted to tell the doctor, I would have. But you're the person who understands my culture and my language and I identify with you. . . . If I knew that you were going to tell the doctor, I wouldn't have told you!" So my colleague at [the first hospital] says, "Don't even put yourself in that position. And don't stay in the exam room or the operating room when the doctor leaves for a minute, because something could happen."

She contrasted this view with that of the community teaching hospital mentioned above, where interpreters (she expects) would likely wonder,

> "Well, but then how could you create trust of a different system?" Maybe . . . it will take the doctor another year to get at information that they need because the patient hasn't felt connected with anyone to feel relaxed and to convey information. And you can still tell the patient that you're part of the health-care team and you must convey information, or "Please don't tell me medical information until we're in the room with the doctor."

This director sees problems with both the black box model and the model that emphasizes strong involvement in patient care. As a result, she advocates a mid-way approach.

Neighborhood Community Clinic: A High-Advocacy Model with an Explicit Social Work Component

The manager of interpreter services at a community health clinic site described her institution as embracing a third model, which, she explained, both welcomes and encourages advocacy on behalf of patients and patients' communities. This manager, the sole interviewee with a master's degree in medical interpretation, explained how surprised she was to discover this model when she first arrived on the job:

> I guess the role of the interpreter here in this clinic is a little more varied than even I was used to. I was very much an interpreter, strictly an interpreter. I'd go in, interpret, and leave. Whereas here there's a lot of social work you don't ever see as a freelancer, because you are staff. So you see a lot of the interpreters helping the patients with documents, or letters that they may get in the mail, or making phone calls for providers, making sure the patient has their medication, things like that. Things that you wouldn't ask an interpreter, a strict interpreter, to do. So I think the role of the interpreter here is a bit different because of that social work aspect.

Although this manager suspects these sorts of social work activities might be more visible to her as a staff member than they were when she worked on a freelance basis, her comments—particularly when compared with those of the other managers interviewed—suggest that it is, indeed, a distinctive feature of this particular community health center.

Although this manager saw much benefit in her clinic's high-advocacy model, she expressed some reservations as well. For example, "coming here it was difficult to see some of the different interpreters doing so much social work because I just felt that the patient might get confused. . . . They may misunderstand the interpreter as giving them the medical advice and not the provider." She explained that this now customary social work aspect has "always been a topic of discussion, you know, whether we should have separate interpreters and separate social workers. Because then the roles will never be mixed up or confused by the patients."

As manager, however, she has promoted the clinic's historically expansive understanding of the interpreter role. She has found that potential new hires are generally open to accepting what she still sees, largely because of her own professional preparation and experience, as added responsibilities. When she interviews job candidates, she explained,

> we tell them that here at the clinic it's a little bit different. . . . You may be asked to call patients when maybe, you know, in another job you wouldn't. But everyone so far has been very willing to take on that aspect. They have that trait in their personality that makes them want to help people, things like that. . . . You know, I think it might change my opinion of whether to hire someone or not if they are just strictly unwilling to be a little bit flexible and help patients in other ways.

As these managers' divergent comments indicate, different health-care institutions hold different expectations of the interpreters they employ, and these differences in expectation are shaped by a variety of factors ranging from technical considerations, such as overall volume of patients per year, to variations in institutional culture, to variations in the professional inclinations and even the personalities of interpreter service managers themselves.

Room for Interpretation? Interpreters' Reflections on the Clinical Triad

The discussion that follows takes a closer look at what happens when the patient-provider pas de deux is transformed into a largely unchoreographed clinical pas de trois. Five of the most prominent themes to emerge in our data are analyzed, including confusion about the differences between clinicians and interpreters; misunderstandings and potential misunderstandings; clinicians' changing views of interpreters; interpreters' frustration with clinicians who "just don't get it"; and the need to teach clinicians how to work with interpreters. All of these themes revolve around one common concern: the persistent ambiguity surrounding the evolving role of medical interpreter in U.S. clinical environments of hyperdiversity.

Differences Between Clinicians and Interpreters

One of the clearest themes to emerge from the interviews conducted is patients' frequent confusion about the nature of the interpreter role. This confusion stems not only from the relative newness of the profession, but also from the absence of a definitive model for everyday interpretive practice and from the common, albeit mistaken, impression that interpreters are themselves clinicians. A Spanish and Portuguese interpreter, for instance, noted that patients do not always understand his role within the clinical interaction. "Some understand perfectly," he said,

> and some don't understand at all. There's a range. . . . I get called "doctor" a lot, even though the first thing I do every time I walk into a room is to identify myself to a patient. I say, "Hello, my name is Mike, I'm a medical interpreter. Everything we say here is confidential." And then some people will respond by saying, "Oh, thanks a lot!" and some respond by saying, "Oh, thank you, Doctor!"

Patients' sense of confidence within the already unequal clinical dynamic can be harmed by mistaken impressions that interpreters are themselves clinicians rather than facilitators whose role is to help the clinical encounter run smoothly.

Other manifestations of this confusion revolve around the role of the interpreter in creating or maintaining a therapeutic alliance. One key issue in this respect involves eye contact. The same interpreter explained, "I've seen entire patient visits where the doctor hasn't looked at the patient, they're just stuck at the computer. Literally, their back is to the patient. Those doctors aren't really going to understand the look on the patient's face." In this interpreter's view, a clinician's lack of engagement creates an added responsibility for him. In such cases, he explained, "I try to compensate by being, you know, extra warm with the patient. I want the patient to feel like they've been cared for, like they have someone in the clinic who cares about them. If it's not going to be the doctor [laughs] then it has to be me." Another Spanish interpreter said that when she tells providers, "You know, it would be best if you made eye contact with the patient instead of with me, and have them make that bond with you rather than with me,' some providers are very open to that and others very quickly forget." Comments like these suggest that clinicians sometimes make the error of outsourcing the social aspects of a clinical encounter to interpreters rather than engaging in direct, if facilitated, interaction with patients themselves.

Misunderstandings and the Boundaries of the Interpreter Role

Another important issue involves misunderstandings and potential misunderstandings about the boundaries of the interpreter role. For instance, some interpreters insist with frustration that their professional mandate to provide a literal translation—no more, no less—prevents them from playing an active role as clarifier or culture broker. In some cases, patients misunderstand a clinical explanation or a set of technical instructions (for instance, about how to take a medication, or how to navigate health care bureaucracy). In other cases, clinicians misunderstand a patient's broader cultural context. A Cape Verdean and Portuguese interpreter, for instance, mentioned that physicians are sometimes perplexed when older patients from Cape Verde are unable to provide their exact date of birth. In such instances, she finds herself educating clinicians about their patients' (and, in this instance, her own) cultural background: "I say, 'I mean, I'm sorry I have to explain to you my culture, my country. It is okay [if] people don't know their age. Especially if you are old.'" In this instance and others like it, an interpreter may intervene by offering cultural knowledge that might help a clinician better understand a patient's broader cultural background. Clarifications like these can help stem discriminatory or prejudicial attitudes that might otherwise be directed at patients. Yet these added interventions are not always seen as inherent to the interpreter role.

Indeed, no clear consensus emerged among interviewees about the appropriate way to handle moments in which a literal translation without clarification would yield misunderstanding or confusion. A few interpreters insisted that providing anything beyond a literal translation is inappropriate. Most, however, believed that interpreters should facilitate clarification either by asking one party to offer more explanation when necessary or by volunteering missing bits of specialized knowledge, whether technical, medical, or cultural. One Spanish interpreter, for instance, said that she can tell when patients "haven't understood a word" and that it is the interpreter's role to intervene "when you see that what is going [on] is going to be misinterpreted, or that the doctor is obviously coming from some place else and isn't really understanding what the patient is saying." In such instances, she continued, "your role as the interpreter is to interrupt and say, 'The interpreter would just like to mention that the patient may not be 100 percent clear on what you just said.' "

Even the manager of interpreter services who advocates something very close to the "invisible conduit" model, and who asks her staff to respect the fact that "the provider is the one in control," nonetheless encourages them to help "bridge the communication." As she elaborated,

> When we see that patients are not asking for clarification, but we can sense that whatever the patient is not asking or what the doctor is not saying can be harmful to the patient. . . . we can kind of like interject without taking over from the provider. And also asking their permission, because the way we will do it [is to] say, "You didn't ask how to take the medication, I'm going to go ahead and ask the question to the provider." And tell the provider, "This is what I told the patient. Can you please go ahead and tell her how to take the medication." Always making sure that we keep both people in the loop. That's the most important thing.

Even at her hospital, which espouses a low-advocacy model of interpretation, a few interpreters mentioned that in certain circumstances they have broken out of their otherwise neutral role to act as patient advocates.

Clinicians at that institution, however, do not necessarily appreciate this sort of intervention. A Japanese interpreter, for instance, described an upsetting situation that arose when she was interpreting on the hospital's obstetric ward. A new mother and her husband had decided well before the birth of their son to have him circumcised before leaving the hospital.

> And then the young doctor came in to circumcise the baby. And before that, [the] doctor started asking [the] patient, "Which of you want to have this baby circumcised?" And she repeated, three or four times, "You're not [a] Jewish person," and "Why do you do this?" . . . until [the] patient started crying.

At that moment, the interpreter felt she had to intervene.

> I said, "Doctor"—this is the first time I ever spoke to a doctor like that— "the patient and husband have decided to circumcise this baby weeks

before, and they know they want to do this. Why do you keep asking? Not once, you ask four times the same question. And [the] patient is very upset." Then the doctor got angry with me . . . because I said my opinion.

Indeed, the incident did not end here; the clinician then asked the interpreter to step outside the room to rebuke her.

Outside the room, [the] doctor said, "You know, you're not supposed to give your opinion. You're supposed to interpret what I say." And I have done that. So she asked my name, and I did do something that [the] interpreter is not supposed to do . . . [because the] patient could not say yes, you know, in a way that convince[d] the doctor. . . . I did have to come back to the office and talk to the director about what happened. And she told me I did fine. So.

For most interviewees—and, furthermore, for their supervisors—it is not only permissible for medical interpreters to play a clarifying role when misunderstandings arise between patients and clinicians, but sometimes imperative to do so.

Clinicians' Changing Views of the Interpreter Role

Not surprisingly, interpreters had much to say about the variety of ways in which clinicians view and interact with them. Some explained that clinicians are now more accustomed to working with interpreters than they were in the past. One experienced Spanish interpreter who had worked in a variety of clinical settings described how she had been shocked by the conduct of the physicians in an academic medical center where she had worked some years ago. There, some of the senior physicians— including high-powered, renowned leaders in their fields—had made little effort to disguise their disdain not only for patients with limited English proficiency and their families, but also for the interpreters hired to help facilitate communication with them. "There was just sort of an arrogance about, 'Why don't you guys [interpreters] all go home and stay out of our hair.' " She laughed, adding, "It was really amazing." Few other interpreters mentioned this level of overt resistance to working with interpreters, although many expressed considerable frustration with physicians who failed to understand the interpreter role.

In general, however, interviewee reflections suggest that clinicians' views of interpreters have changed considerably in recent decades. The manager of interpreter services at one academic medical center, for instance, explained that over the past two decades, interpretation has come to be viewed at her institution "more as a profession and part of the medical team than . . . before." This shift, which is partly a function of the region's growing hyperdiversity, holds deep clinical significance.

Not only does it imply a growing recognition that providers cannot do their jobs adequately if language barriers impede communication, but it also implies a parallel recognition that ad hoc alternatives to professional interpretation are no longer satisfactory. In the past, this manager explained,

> providers viewed the interpreters more kind of like an intruder, being in the middle of an encounter, rather than a working partner. And now they do understand that in order to have better communication and to have better outcomes, they really need to work with someone that is professional and that has the right background and the knowledge to do a good interpretation.

A Spanish interpreter echoed these sentiments on the basis of her own experience. Most providers, she said,

> learn to accept the interpreter as part of the medical team. So they work very well with us most of the time. Again, every so often you'll find someone who will constantly interrupt, and any time the patient says something, they don't let him finish a complete phrase. They're halfway through, and they say, "What are they saying? What are they saying?" You have to tell them, "Well, if you let me listen, I could tell you." [laughs] But again, that's not most of the time. Most of the time it works out very well.

Although clinicians may evince a growing appreciation for professional interpreters, appreciation and recognition do not necessarily translate into a clear understanding of the specific tasks that interpreters can and cannot—or will and will not—perform.

Frustration with Clinicians Who "Just Don't Get It"

For a number of interpreters interviewed, a key challenge remains the fact that some clinicians "just don't get it." As a U.S.-born Spanish interpreter at an academic medical center explained,

> We're trained to try and promote the most direct relationship possible between the patient and the provider, because that's the main relationship. But what providers tend to do is instead of looking at a patient and saying, "Oh, so how are you doing, Mrs. Fernandez? How is your pain?" and I'll repeat the same thing in Spanish—instead of doing that, they turn and look at me and say, "OK, so I just need you to check with him how his pain is, [and so on]" . . . And they want to look at me the whole time and not at the patient. So it's almost like we're talking about the patient. As if we were two doctors talking about the patient, with the patient actually standing there in the room. . . . Some people, they just don't get it.

For this interpreter, this dynamic is disheartening and possibly damaging. It destroys the myth of invisibility that this interpreter regards as the hallmark of her profession. In addition, it marks her as a socially present stakeholder in the interaction and aligns her with the clinician in a manner that risks leaving the patient feeling trapped in a two-against-one situation.

This is but one among many instances in which interviewees expressed frustration with clinicians who just don't get it. Another Spanish interpreter, for example, described how one doctor treated her like she was ignorant when she sought to provide what she understood to be her professional mandate: a literal translation.

> I've been in an interpretation where a patient was saying, "I went to the doctor because my baby had a high fever, and they put a needle in the back, and they took some fluid." And the doctor turned around and said, "Well, that's a lumbar puncture." And I said, "Thank you very much, I know that, but the patient didn't know that. So I'm interpreting what the patient is saying. I'm not here to show you that I know all these medical terms, because that's not the point. It's not about me over there, knowing or not knowing."

In other words, not only might patients misconstrue interpreters as being improperly aligned with health-care providers, but providers may also project their views of patients—including disparaging or discriminatory views—onto interpreters because it is they, and not the patients, with whom physicians can communicate directly.

Interestingly, these frustrations emerged consistently across health-care institutions despite divergent understandings of the interpreter role. For example, the interpreter services manager at the first academic medical center said, "The most frustrating is when they [staff interpreters] work with providers that don't know how to work with an interpreter. And then that makes them feel very frustrated." Some providers "are asking us to do a lot of things that we're not supposed to be doing." For instance, providers will sometimes say, "consent the patient, I'll be back' [that is, obtain the patient's informed consent for a medical procedure]. We shouldn't be doing that." At other times, clinicians will say,

> "Just tell me the important things and omit the things that are not important." No thank you very much, we're not doing that. You figure out what is important and what is not important. So that can be frustrating because we have . . . a role that we have to fulfill when we go to different encounters. And it gets disrupted when you're working with someone who doesn't know how you work.

The manager at the second academic medical center also noted that some providers have unreasonable expectations of interpreters:

> So, for example, a provider may get up . . . and say, "Can you just find out if she's had any history of this and that, and then ask her this and this," and then leave. And that's not how interpreting works. I'm not a provider, so you know . . . It always has to be a three-way conversation. So sometimes it's difficult to not have providers just get up and leave you there, you know, kind of doing a part of their job to kind of make things go faster. Because we're just not prepared for any of that.

Regardless of institutional setting, interviewees consistently expressed frustration with clinicians who misunderstand the role of the interpreter. In some cases, misunderstandings occur when clinicians project emotions, attitudes, or stereotypes onto interpreters rather than try to understand their patients with an interpreter's assistance. In other instances, misunderstandings arise when clinicians ask interpreters to function like clinicians by engaging in tasks that are beyond their training and expertise.

One Spanish interpreter hypothesized that some clinicians have difficulty working with interpreters because the language barrier between them and their patients leaves them feeling intimidated or insecure:

> This is just my impression, but I feel like some of it comes from insecurity. Like, kind of almost like they're intimidated because they can't speak the person's language. Because sometimes I've noticed . . . that when I do tell them, you know, "You can feel free to look at the patient, talk to the patient," . . . then there is kind of more understanding happening between them and the patient, and they look at each others' eyes and they say, "Oh, okay, do you understand the plan, Mrs. So-and-So?" and they say, "Yes."

In cases like these, granting clinicians explicit permission to engage their patients directly can have a liberating effect. For this interpreter, she has found that afterwards "the provider turns to me and says, 'Oh, thank you so much,' you know, almost like they're grateful. Almost like they feel relieved, because maybe they feel intimidated. . . . They feel almost like being on the outside, like shut out. And so not speaking directly to the patient is a way of kind of alienating the patient, or fighting back against that somehow."

If this interpreter's hunch is correct, then one possible solution to the myriad moments of frustration recounted by interviewees might lie in so simple an intervention as a brief training session for clinicians offering practical instruction and role-playing exercises designed to improve their confidence in working with interpreters.

The Need for Clinician Training

Indeed, this is precisely what the director of interpreter services at one academic medical center proposed: a "mandatory health-care provider training on how to work with interpreters" involving role play in which providers can "see an actual interpreter triage. See how it works, show them what to do or what not to do. And it wouldn't have to be more than an hour. An hour out of everyone's medical career is not going to kill them." In her view, such an intervention would be valuable for clinicians at all career stages, but it would be especially helpful for younger clinicians and clinicians in training. "Our doctors here, for the most part, our nurses . . . many are probably pretty good. Some aren't but it's not their fault, and especially the older ones, it's hard to change how they work after forty years. . . . There's a better shot for newer folks to get a little more training. But definitely there's training missing. And I don't think that it would have to be horribly extensive, but there isn't a formal place for it."

Not only does institutional pressure to use clinicians' time efficiently stand in the way of developing formal training sessions on how to work with interpreters, but a second constraint stands in the way as well: the unequal power dynamic between clinicians and interpreters and between medical units and interpreter units within health care centers. Although some interpreters described patient education as part of their professional mandate, the parallel notion of provider education made several interpreters uncomfortable because it implied a sense of stepping on the doctor's toes or otherwise questioning (or threatening) their expertise. Without underestimating the significance of this power dynamic, it is important to cast a clear light on this common if paradoxical situation. How can we make sense of the fact that substantial resources are invested in hiring and employing professional medical interpreters, and yet clinicians—the health-care staff with whom interpreters will work most closely—are exempted from the kind of training that could help make their interpreted clinical encounters proceed smoothly?

Conclusion

As new patterns of immigration and growing hyperdiversity transform the demographic profile of United States communities, health-care institutions are becoming increasingly attuned to the need for medical interpreter services. New legal statutes combined with growing recognition that ad hoc interpreters offer only a partial and problematic solution have strengthened many health-care institutions' commitment to integrating professional medical interpreters into health-care teams.

A number of insights emerge from these findings. First, although the role of the medical interpreter is currently undergoing a process of professionalization, it is still open-ended, nonstandardized, and undefined. Because no standardized training curriculum and no universally recognized certificate or diploma exist, interpreters' training experiences vary considerably. In some cases, interpreters have undergone no professional training whatsoever (although the administrators interviewed for this study now express a preference for hiring professionally trained interpreters). Not only do prevailing models of interpretation vary—for instance, from the invisible conduit model at one end of the spectrum, to the model of the culture broker–patient advocate on the other—but different health-care institutions also expect very different things from their staff interpreters. At some institutions, for instance, interpreters are strongly discouraged from interacting with patients outside of the clinical encounter in any way. At others, interpreters are told before they are hired that their jobs will involve a substantial social work component.

Second, as the interview data presented here clearly illustrate, the core myth of interpreter invisibility that animates the models of medical interpretation promoted by professional organizations and training programs is quite distant from the everyday reality of interpretive practice. Contrary to functioning as invisible machines or ghosts, interpreters are always and inevitably social actors. They must make numerous small choices in the course of their work—for example, to sit with the patient in the waiting room or not; to chitchat before the doctor enters the room or not; to insist that a misunderstanding be clarified or not. These choices can profoundly affect a clinician's ability to obtain an accurate and complete medical history; the development of a therapeutic alliance; a patient's level of trust in the clinician and the health-care institution; the overall process of diagnosis, treatment, and patient involvement in the treatment process; and ultimately health-care outcomes.

Third, the growing emphasis on training interpreters to work with clinicians without investing in the parallel component of this process carries some irony. Certain clinicians are finding it difficult to work effectively within a transformed, now-triadic clinical space. Some senior clinicians, for instance, are reluctant to adapt after a long professional career, and, as one Spanish interpreter said, "There's always a small percentage of people who I guess were in the wrong career, you know. They just don't have very much patience." Overall, however, most of the interpreters interviewed report not only that clinicians generally are willing to adapt to their presence and the complications it entails, but also that clinicians seem to be more comfortable working with interpreters when all parties involved understand the rules of this unconventional form of social interaction. These insights lead us to ask a crucial question: why are health-care institutions investing so much of their limited resources in building whole new departments—interpreter service units—without streamlining the entry of these units' staff into their institutions as a whole?

As one manager of interpreter services explained, the integration of interpreters into the clinical dynamic involves a learning curve for all parties involved. In order for this pas de trois to work effectively, both patients and clinicians must be prepared to adapt and even compromise. "Obviously, it's more cumbersome" to involve an interpreter than to communicate directly in a shared language. To make things work, she explained, "the doctor has to give up some control . . . everybody has to give up a little bit." After all, she pointed out, "you could get a really bad doctor who speaks your language. . . . Just because a doctor speaks your language doesn't mean you're going to get good care. And that's the truth in English just as much as it is in Chinese, or Somali, or any other language."

Notes

1. Thanks are due to Miki Cohen Moskowitz and Elisabeth Poorman for conducting these interviews and for their valuable contributions to an early version of this chapter.
2. Some interpreters work in more than one language. Other languages for which interpretation services were available at study sites included Russian, Italian, French, Vietnamese, Khmer, Cantonese, and Mandarin.
3. Increasing levels of LEP are related to rates of immigration to the United States and the increase in households in which English is not the primary language spoken. Between 1980 and 2007, the percentage of U.S. residents who spoke a language other than English at home increased nearly twofold, from 11 percent to 20 percent (U.S. Census Bureau 2011).

References

ACORN. 2004. *Speaking the Language of Care: Language Barriers to Hospital Access in America's Cities.* Washington, D.C.: Association of Community Organizations for Reform Now.

Alexieva, Bistra. 2002. "A Typology of Interpreter-Mediated Events." In *The Interpreting Studies Reader,* edited by Franz Pöchhacker and Miriam Shlesinger. London: Routledge.

Angelelli, Claudia V. 2004a. *Medical Interpreting and Cross-Cultural Communication.* Cambridge: Cambridge University Press.

———. 2004b. *Revising the Interpreter's Role: A Study of Conference, Court, and Medical Interpreters in Canada, Mexico, and the United States.* Amsterdam: John Benjamins.

Baker, David, Risa Hayes, and Julia Puebla Fortier. 1998. "Interpreter Use and Satisfaction with Interpersonal Aspects of Care for Spanish-Speaking Patients." *Medical Care* 36(10): 1461–470.

Bot, Hanneke. 2005. *Dialogue Interpreting in Mental Health,* vol. 19, *Utrecht Studies in Language and Communication.* Amsterdam: Rodopi.

Chen, Alice Hm, Mara K. Youdelman, and Jamie Brooks. 2007. "The Legal Framework for Language Access in Healthcare Settings: Title VI and Beyond." *Journal of General Internal Medicine* 22(supplement 2): 362–67.

Davidson, Brad. 2000. "The Interpreter as Institutional Gatekeeper: The Social-Linguistic Role of Interpreters in Spanish-English Medical Discourse." *Journal of Sociolinguistics* 4(3): 379–405.

Drennan, Gerald, and Leslie Swartz. 2002. "The Paradoxical Use of Interpreting in Psychiatry." *Social Science & Medicine* 54(12): 1853–866.

Dye, Eva. 2001. "Use of Translation Cards to Increase Communication with Non-English-Speaking Families in the NICU." *Neonatal Network* 20(7): 25–29.

Fernandez, Alicia, Dean Schillinger, Kevin Grumbach, Anne Rosenthal, Anita L. Stewart, Frances Wang, and Eliseo J. Pérez-Stable. 2004. "Physician Language Ability and Cultural Competence: An Exploratory Study of Communication with Spanish-Speaking Patients." *Journal of General and Internal Medicine* 19(2004): 167–74.

Flores, Glenn, M. Barton Laws, Sandra J. Mayo, Barry Zuckerman, Milagros Abreu, Leonardo Medina, and Eric J. Hardt. 2003. "Errors in Medical Interpretation and Their Potential Clinical Consequences in Pediatric Encounters." *Pediatrics* 111(1): 6–14.

Haffner, Linda. 1992. "Translation Is Not Enough: Interpreting in a Medical Setting." *Western Journal of Medicine* 157(3): 255–59.

Hampers, Louis C., and Jennifer E. McNulty. 2002. "Professional Interpreters and Bilingual Physicians in a Pediatric Emergency Department." *Archives of Pediatric Adolescent Medicine* 156(11): 1108–113.

Jacobs, Elizabeth A., Alice Hm Chen, Leah S. Karliner, Niels Agger-Gupta, and Sunita Mutha. 2006. "The Need for More Research on Language Barriers in Health Care: A Proposed Research Agenda." *The Millbank Quarterly* 84(1): 111–33.

Jacobs, Elizabeth A., Diane S. Lauderdale, David Meltzer, Jeanette M. Shorey, Wendy Levinson, and Ronald A. Thisted. 2001. "Impact of Interpreter Services on Delivery of Healthcare to Limited-English-Proficient Patients." *Journal of General Internal Medicine* 16(7): 468–74.

Kaplan, Sherrie H., Sheldon Greenfield, and John E. Ware. 1989. "Assessing the Effects of Physician Interactions on the Outcomes of Chronic Disease." *Medical Care* 27(3): S110–S127.

Kaufert, Joseph, and Robert Putsch. 1997. "Communication Through Interpreters in Healthcare: Ethical Dilemmas Arising from Differences in Class, Culture, Language, and Power." *Journal of Clinical Ethics* 8(1): 71–87.

Kopczynski, Andrej. 1994. "Quality in Conference Interpreting: Some Pragmatic Problems." In *Translation Studies: An Interdiscipline,* edited by Mary Snell-Hornby, Franz Pöchhacker, and Klaus Kaindl. Amsterdam: John Benjamins.

Mayer, Gloria G., and Michael Villaire. 2007. *Health Literacy in Primary Care: A Clinician's Guide.* New York: Springer.

Miller, Kenneth, Zoe L. Martell, Linda Pazdirek, Melissa Caruth, and Diana Lopez. 2007. "The Role of Interpreters in Psychotherapy with Refugees: An Exploratory Study." *American Journal of Orthopsychiatry* 75(1): 27–39.

Moreno, Maria R., Regina Otero-Sabogal, and Jeffrey Newman. 2007. "Assessing Dual-Role Staff-Interpreter Linguistic Competency in an Integrated Healthcare System." *Journal of General Internal Medicine* 22(supplement 2): 331–35.

National Health Law Program and National Council on Interpreting in Health Care. 2007. *Language Services Resource Guide for Health Care Providers.* Washington, D.C.: National Health Law Program.

National Health Law Program and The Access Project. 2003. *Language Services Action Kit: Interpreter Services in Health Care Settings for People with Limited English Proficiency.* Available at: http://www.accessproject.org/adobe/language_services_action_kit.pdf (accessed June 24, 2011).

Office of Minority Health. 2001. "National Standards for Culturally and Linguistically Appropriate Services in Health Care Final Report." Washington: U.S. Department of Health and Human Services. Available at: http://www.omhrc.gov/templates/content.aspx?ID=87 (accessed June 24, 2011).

Perkins, Jane, and Mara Youdelman. 2006. *Summary of State Law Requirements: Addressing Language Needs in Health Care.* Washington, D.C.: National Health Law Program.

Perkins, Jane, Mara Youdelman, and Doreen Wong. 2003. *Ensuring Linguistic Access in Health Care Settings: Legal Rights and Responsibilities.* Washington, D.C.: National Health Law Program.

Prince, C. 1986. "Hablando Con el Doctor: Communication Problems between Doctors and Their Spanish-Speaking Patients." Ph.D. diss., Stanford University.

Roy, Cynthia. 2002. "The Problem with Definitions, Descriptions, and the Role of Metaphors of Interpreters." In *The Interpreting Studies Reader,* edited by Franz Pöchhacker and Miriam Shlesinger. London: Routledge.

Sampson, Alyssa. 2006. *Language Services Resource Guide for Health Care Providers.* Los Angeles: National Health Law Program.

Shin, Hyon B., with Rosalind Bruno. 2003. *Language Use and English-Speaking Ability: 2000.* Washington: U.S. Census Bureau.

Takka, G. 1991. *Differential Access to Health Care of Latino Children in the Hispanic Health and Nutrition Examination Survey.* Palo Alto, Calif.: Stanford University Press.

Timmins, C. L. 2002. "The Impact of Language Barriers on the Health Care of Latinos in the United States: A Review of the Literature." *Journal of Midwifery and Women's Health* 47(2): 80–96.

Tribe, Rachel, and Hitesh Rayal, eds. 2002. *Working with Interpreters in Mental Health.* New York: Routledge.

U.S. Census Bureau. 2010. "American Community Survey, Detailed Languages Spoken at Home and Ability to Speak English for the Population 5 Years and Over for the United States." Available at: http://go.usa.gov/bsl (accessed June 24, 2011).

———. 2011. "Table 2: Languages Spoken at Home: 1980, 1990, 2000, and 2007." Available at: http://www.census.gov/hhes/socdemo/language/data/acs/appendix.html (accessed June 24, 2011).

Wadensjö, Cecilia. 1998. *Interpreting as Interaction.* New York: Addison Wesley Longman.

Woloshin, Steven, Nina A. Bickell, Lisa M. Schwartz, Francesca Gany, and H. Gilbert Welch. 1995. "Language Barriers in Medicine in the United States." *Journal of the American Medical Association* 273(9): 724–28.

Woloshin, Steven, Lisa M. Schwartz, Steven J. Katz, and H. Gilbert Welch. 1997. "Is Language a Barrier to the Use of Preventive Services?" *Journal of General Internal Medicine* 12(8): 472–77.

Chapter 4

Praying Along:
Interfaith Chaplaincy
and the Politics of Translation

LISA STEVENSON

"I THINK I'm lucky," an interfaith chaplain at a major research hospital in Boston said. "Because I get to talk about things like feelings and faith. And prayer. And all of those questions that are hard, like, 'What's the meaning of life?' and 'Why is this terrible thing happening?' And I'm allowed to do that and I get paid to do that. And so part of my role here is to give people permission to speak about these things. I remember one neurologist [who] said, 'That mother was talking to spirits! Can you believe that?' And I said, 'So? I do that every day. It's called prayer.'"

The chaplain makes a series of strategic distinctions, the first being that she is paid to ask about the meaning of life, whereas doctors are paid to "maintain life" (Weber 1948.) The equation of prayer with talking to spirits was also a strategic move on the chaplain's part: she wanted to convince the neurologist that the mother's seemingly bizarre behavior was not so different from her own, and in so doing, she hoped to make discursive room ("the permission to speak about these things") for alternative religious practices within the hospital. Prayer has its place in an American hospital, but does talking to spirits?

Yet the chaplain's implicit nominalism—her belief that the two practices in question are fundamentally the same, distinguished only by different names (*prayer* and *talking to spirits*)—raises several important anthropological questions. What is the nature of human difference—those practices, beliefs, and values that constitute what anthropologists call otherness? Should such difference be conceived in nominalist terms—as a

94

question of the language we use to describe our worlds? Or are there differences that resist translation—differences in the face of which language and translation, in one way or another, fails us? The answers to such questions are never innocent and the stakes for a chaplain in asserting the equivalence of prayer and talking to spirits will be addressed in what follows.

Ironically, it is the anthropologist's concept of culture, as popularized and incorporated into discourses of multiculturalism, that has allowed this nominalistic view of culture as transparently translatable to gain traction. From Franz Boas forward, the culture concept was an important attempt to combat racism and to dismantle the notion of human hierarchy. Thus, early anthropologists wanted to show that alien cultures were in fact understandable—that is, translatable into the terms of Western culture.[1] No longer saddled by the evolutionary matrix in which indigenous peoples were somehow less evolved than Western peoples, culture groups could be celebrated for their different ways of adapting to their environment, different religious, and social practices. Yet, by the 1980s, multiculturalism's emphasis on the equivalence of cultures resulted in a further entrenchment of translation as an unproblematic act of inscribing the other in the terms of the self. Today "culture" has been incorporated into the clinic in ways that make many anthropologists uneasy. The notion of translatability has been taken to an extreme: culture can be reduced (to be easily translatable) to a "core set of beliefs about illness owing to fixed ethnic traits. Cultural competency often becomes a series of 'do's and don'ts' that define how to treat a patient of a given ethnic background" (Kleinman and Benson 2006, 1673).

In this chapter I trace the way, in the context of interfaith chaplaincy in one Boston area hospital, religious difference gets subsumed under the culture concept and the possibility of translation comes to be taken for granted. My critique of this use of the culture concept is not meant to diminish the considerable dangers inherent to holding the opposite view—namely, that particular religious or cultural practices are untranslatable. Such dangers are manifest in, for example, the way suicide bombers are understood in the West. Their actions are framed as so morally reprehensible, even unthinkable, that attempts to understand what leads to such acts of violence are rarely made (Asad 2007; Hage 2003; Murray 2006). Instead of arguing that cultural translation is either unproblematic or impossible, I want to suggest that the act of translation, conceived as a *practice of the self*,[2] offers a productive way to engage cultural and religious difference. It opens up the possibility that the self will be transformed or converted in the process of that translation.

I came to investigate the work of hospital chaplaincy in a roundabout way. Charged with finding out whether culturally specific services actually make a difference in American health care, I began to interview the hospital chaplains only after several nurses and social workers offered it as a good example of the cultural services their hospital provided. I was initially struck by the ease with which my interlocutors substituted religion for culture—that is, I had asked about culturally specific services and they directed me to the chaplaincy.

Then, as I began to interview the chaplains, I was surprised by the way religious difference, such as the difference between prayer and talking to spirits, was repeatedly articulated through the concept of culture. What I came to understand is that religion, to make itself palatable to hospital bureaucracies and medical discourse, has had to reformulate itself in cultural and therefore translatable terms. That is, religion is rarely described as an alternate healing system, a powerful political and moral force, or even a path to universal truth. In fact, it can be argued that "religion" is being replaced with what one chaplain I interviewed called "the culture of religiosity."

The idea that there is such a thing as the culture of religiosity highlights our assumption that all religions have something important in common. But even this idea—that religions are comparable—has an important and interesting genealogy. Talal Asad has argued that the very idea that there could be a universal definition of religion, against which different religions could be compared or through which they could be translated, enjoys a very specific, and Christian, history (1993b). In the face of the rising power of science in the sixteenth and seventeenth century, the Church came to define religion "as a set of propositions to which believers gave assent, and which could therefore be judged and compared between different religions and as against natural science" (41). By focusing narrowly on religious belief (embedded in a set of propositions) as opposed to a set of practices, the Church no longer had to compete with the astounding efficacy of science. Distinguishing secular scientific practice from religious belief thus maintained a place for the authority of the Church.

In American hospitals today, the stakes are somewhat different. *Religion* (universally conceived) is vying for a place within the hospital bureaucracy—religion seeks to be incorporated into the medical model of care. If the goal is to assimilate religion into the hospital bureaucracy, (to "give people permission to speak about such things") the question becomes less about the comparison of religious belief systems, or about staking out a domain for religion in the face of science, as it is about the commensuration of one religion to another and then the insertion of religion into medical discourse. By commensuration I mean the process by which two terms are rendered equivalent, or in the case cited, the way in which otherness is rewritten in terms of the self. Differences between religions (what under the model of translation might remain untranslatable) become inconsequential. The emphasis shifts to a universal human need for spirituality in whatever form it takes. For hospital bureaucrats, spirituality becomes a black box for a kind of "psycho-social" need (Lee 2002, 346) that is never fully elucidated.

Religion on the Front Sheet

In 1998 the U.S. Joint Commission on Accreditation of Healthcare Organizations (JCAHO) adopted standards for the provision of "adequate spiritual care" that were later made an accreditation requirement for American hospitals (Lee 2002). Although JCAHO "first considered religion and spirituality in 1969, the guidelines were significantly revised in the 1990s when the religious-spiritual care of patients was framed as a right, addressed under the heading of Patient Rights (Cadge, Freese, and Christakis 2008). Today, as one nurse in a Boston-area hospital put it, "Your religion is on the front sheet." This means that in the admissions process, "nursing is required to document whether a patient has religious preferences and if they want to be visited by the chaplaincy department during their stay."

Before the 1990s and JCAHO's explicit interest in the spiritual needs of patients, chaplaincy was a faith-specific vocation with Roman Catholic priests, Protestant ministers, and Jewish rabbis working alongside each other but rarely interacting. The current head of one chaplaincy department described the chaplains of that era as lone ranger figures—unpaid and largely invisible in the hospital bureaucratic structures. In the 1990s, a shift occurred that led to the creation of what is called the interfaith chaplain. This was also the moment when hospitals began to pay chaplains a salary and to see them as hospital employees.

This concept of interfaith chaplain heralded a whole new way of conceiving of the chaplain's work: hospital administrations began to talk in terms of the spiritual needs of the patient, and the chaplaincy was understood to provide a spiritual service. This has been conceptualized as a shift from the religiously based theological practice of hospital chaplaincy to a secularized and professional practice (Lee 2002). As the director of chaplaincy in one Boston-area hospital explained to me, with a staff of eight full-time chaplains, four part-time chaplains, and six or seven per-diem chaplains, "we are literally one of the departments in [the] patient care services chain." Chaplains, still performing some faith-specific duties, are each assigned to hospital wards according to a medical specialty—not their faith tradition. Thus one chaplain is in charge of neurology wards, another pediatrics, another psychiatry, and so on.

As chaplaincy came to be refigured as just another service the hospital provides, the range of religious backgrounds represented also expanded. Instead of having a few priests and one rabbi to call on, the chaplaincy includes members of a variety of Protestant traditions, a Muslim imam, and a Buddhist practitioner. Representatives of Jehovah's Witness, Christian Science, Mormons, and Hindu Swamis can be brought in on an as-needed basis. Yet even as the number of "faith perspectives" represented multiplies, the idea that all faiths are equal becomes increasingly entrenched. There is a way in which the different religions or faith perspectives are conceived as so many (equivalent) options from which the patient can choose, although that choice is ultimately unimportant.

In fact, I am arguing that the only way religion can be legible in the hospital setting is if it is no longer understood as a potentially incongruous healing practice, or as a divergent political power structure, or even as a different ontological system. Instead, it must be subsumed by the culture concept, which in some sense renders religious belief and practice as a harmless, interesting, but inessential form of difference.

A director of chaplaincy from another Boston-area hospital spoke of this shift with some resignation: "[Chaplaincy] is now becoming, in some ways, removed more from religion per se. It speaks of this new cultural thing—which is something I have great difficulty with—which is called spirituality. . . . What's happening now in chaplaincy is you're finding people who are being trained to come from different religious traditions, or *non*-religious traditions, wanting to take this spiritualism . . . and put it into practice."

In the remainder of this chapter I trace, in a necessarily preliminary way, the way in which religious belief is being subsumed by this culture of religiosity that commensurates different religions (prayer and talking to spirits are "the same thing") to make them palatable to the rationalized bureaucratic world of the hospital that attends to the "universal" suffering subject (on the notion of universal suffering, see Young 1996). This celebration of the culture concept leads to a paradoxical situation—one in which respecting difference often means effacing it through a process of commensuration in which the other is made intelligible to the self. Difference is literally absorbed into sameness. Prayer is talking to spirits.

Elizabeth Povinelli's version of this particular liberal dilemma is that representatives of "radical worlds" are called on to "be other so that we will not ossify, but be in such a way that we are not undone, that is make yourself doable for us" (2001, 329). Continuing with our example, to be "doable" means to be able to say, "Your talking to spirits is really harmless; it's just like my prayer." Ultimately, however, this means that liberal ideology and practice are not themselves commensurate. As liberal subjects, we want to see and value all difference, but some difference is just too difficult, some differences are not ultimately doable. Undoable difference marks the limits of recognition, the moments when liberal ideology diverges from liberal practice. Thus though hospital staff celebrate the Catholic desire to baptize babies in the neonatal intensive care unit (NICU), or bring prayer mats to Muslim patients in the psychiatric ward, the Haitian woman who refuses a transfusion because she believes her child has been cursed is less doable for her caregivers. That is, religion must exist in the hospital in such a way that it neither threatens the epistemology nor reach of biomedicine. Spirituality comes to be understood as a kind of placebo effect (compare Hahn and Kleinman 1983), and is assimilated to vaguely defined notions of the importance of psycho-social care. So when the Haitian woman refused a blood transfusion, a Catholic priest was called in to try to bring the woman into line with biomedical practice. "Even the Pope had a transfusion," he told her.

Although hospital administrators want to be the kind of people that respect and accommodate difference, ultimately it's still a matter of the patient's having "correct belief"—a belief that will help prevent and cure disease (on the question of correct belief and a discussion of the problem of belief in medical anthropology, see Good 1994b). Religion's difference from medicine must be both celebrated and, in practice, insignificant.

To a large degree, at least in the hospital, the chaplain's ability to escape this liberal dilemma—through, for example, providing an alternative articulation of the stakes of healing—has been diminished. There are also high stakes for chaplains in refusing to be doable for hospital staff—they risk expulsion from the hospital. This fear of being "out of a job" if your religion isn't doable for hospital staff is something I discuss later. But first I want to call attention a very important point that could get lost in a discussion of the way religion is made commensurate to hospital forms. In the slippage between the discourse of religiosity and the day-to-day practice of chaplaincy in the hospital there are in fact moments where chaplaincy can indeed provide a space for something else, something beyond an unswerving attention to the health, or "life" as Max Weber (1948) would have it, of the body.

Praying Along

I had the opportunity to accompany one chaplain on her rounds of the locked psychiatric ward in her hospital. The first patient we visited, a woman in her fifties, was sitting absently on a chair across from the hospital bed, worrying a pamphlet between her fingers. Susanna, the chaplain, knew from the patient's chart that she had struggled for years with severe depression. She also knew the woman was Roman Catholic. Susanna was Protestant. Susanna sat down on the bed facing the woman, hunching her shoulders, as if to make her presence less threatening.

"When you are feeling depressed, does your faith help?" she asked gently. As an answer the woman showed us the leaflet she was holding in her hands, which was filled with Catholic prayers for different occasions.

"Oh yes," said Susanna excitedly, "and you know what I have? People always like these." She pulled from her binder a series of glossy cards with pictures of various saints and corresponding prayer. "Would you like to have one of these? Which one?" The patient became animated and, scanning the cards quickly, she chose one with a picture of the Virgin Mary.

"That's the one I collected as a little girl," she said happily. "When I was in grade school the Sisters would always let us choose one of these when we did good work. I had a lot of them."

"I bet you did," laughed Susanna. Then she asked her if she would like to pray. Together they read the prayer printed on the card, one the patient seemed to know by heart.

Later I ask Susanna about her experience as a Protestant chaplain handing out Catholic prayer cards. "Was I praying when I read that prayer?" she muses. "I was praying along. Would it have been more authentic if I had prayed spontaneously? Probably. Probably yes."[3]

No Atheists in Foxholes

Another way to address the challenge of interfaith chaplaincy, the challenge of how best to "pray along" with patients is to invoke the universality of the suffering subject. When I asked a rabbi about the cultural issues he faced when attending to the needs of people of different faiths and cultures within the hospital, he reframed the issue in terms of a universal humanity. "Mostly, people just are glad to have someone to listen to," he told me. "There's something about being in a hospital that transcends cultural issues because there are no atheists in foxholes. . . . They want to be with somebody else, whether or not they want to talk to God." The same rabbi repeated to me several times the mantra of hospital chaplaincy: "Don't just do something—stand there!" And when I followed this rabbi on his rounds what most surprised me—and made me the most uncomfortable—was how little he said during his visits. He would enter a room, introduce himself and then stand there, leaning slightly forward. "That's sort of the simplest version of our chaplaincy," he explained to me in an interview. We show up as people, and we might also bring God if they want, but the most important thing is that they want another human being to be concerned about them." Suffering breaks down the barriers between people, difference between religions become insignificant, the universality of the suffering subject is foregrounded.

Yet at the same time as many of the chaplains were emphasizing the way culture ceases to matter in the face of profound suffering, they were providing me with nuanced examples of the way they attend to a patient's cultural *habitus*—if only so that they can get "beyond" it to the patient's underlying humanity. Thus the Jewish chaplain describes his way of "being present" to the patient who is suffering:

> That you don't, you don't say anything specifically, and in that you don't give any cultural response, your response is presence, and then it only matters about little things that aren't so little, like distance. How far away do you sit from a person? Do you sit very close? You try to take cues from what they tell you to do. Do you sit down or stand up the whole time? Some people really want you stand up the whole time and be in an official role, some people want you to sit down and relax, and you want— you're always reading that.

Another chaplain, a priest who was originally from Nigeria, points out that this bodily language, of sitting near, of standing up, of coming closer or going farther, are precisely what is cultural about the interaction. He says,

> So one time I went to see a white lady on my floor, and she wanted confession. And I sat down, I said, "OK, let's start." And she says, "I can't!" And I say, "Why not?" And she says, "I need to have the screen, so I don't see you," because she was brought up in a time in the history of Catholic practice where to go to Confession there has to be a screen so the Confessor won't see you. And she was eighty-two. And I said, "Can I turn my back so you don't see my face?" And she said, "I can't! I still see you."

However, when the priest tried to hear the confession of a young school-aged boy in his parish, he had the opposite problem. The boy came and knelt before him in the confessional (which had a screen) but was not saying anything. The chaplain recounted their conversation:

> "Are you there?"
> "I am."
> "Can you start?"
> "I can't!"
> "Why not?"
> "Because I can't see you."

The chaplain explained to me, "You see? He was brought up in the age of face-to-face, like you see a doctor face-to-face. So when the screen was there, he just couldn't do it."

For this chaplain the physical discomfort of both the old woman and the young boy point to cultural differences that are experienced in the body. It is the body that may actually betray the chaplain's desire to be a good liberal subject always willing to accept and respect such forms of difference. The Catholic chaplain spoke movingly of the way his own body would give him away if he attempted to support someone in a situation that radically contradicted his beliefs. He described being called into an abortion on the grounds of genetic abnormality, something his faith does not condone.

> So sometimes it's a struggle for me; will my going in there mean that I am endorsing the practice, or will going in there mean that I will allow someone whose conscience is hurting to experience the comfort and mercy of God? And they are hurting. So sometimes I live with that ethical dilemma. . . .
>
> It's very, very difficult. If I go in, is it scandalous, supporting people in doing something that my religion specifically says is wrong? And when that feeling is extremely very strong, I may say, "I am sorry, I just cannot do it." As where I respect my own belief, there are things I cannot do. If somebody else is willing to do it, that's fine; because if I go into the situation, I start sharing my own belief, that person might think that I am accusing [them] of not doing the right thing, instead of my presence easing their pain. You see the point? Even my body will communicate this discomfort and disapproval, and they will pick up. So from my face, and my body. I will not be in a position to comfort, to provide a caring and compassionate care.

This chaplain showed great sensitivity to the small and unexpected ways human beings may differ from another, and the ways we express our discomfort with that difference. In contemporary chaplaincy this difference is rarely judged. It is accepted. This is in line, of course, with what I have outlined—the liberal notion of how to live with difference and how to understand culture. We accept, explore, and enjoy differences. As religious beliefs are subsumed by the culture concept, religions also become commensurable and are thus excluded from judgment. But this very sensitive chaplain, who believes that abortion is wrong, struggles profoundly. Part of his struggle is whether he should take a cultural or religious view of the matter. Sometimes he goes and comforts the patient, knowing that she has a different (cultural) view of what has just happened. Other times he just can't make himself. However, he says, "if somebody else is willing to do it, that's fine." There is no judgment being made about others who can comfort the woman without compunction. Even if their beliefs and practices are diametrically opposed, still, "it's fine."

Belief in Belief

But perhaps the chaplain who best embodied this move toward a "culture of religiosity"—which presumes to be able to move beyond the specificity of particular faith traditions—was the chaplain at one Boston-area hospital who listed her faith tradition as the Ethical Culture Movement (ECM). ECM eschews any deity and calls itself "a democratic community and spiritual home for those who seeks a rational, compassionate approach to life." This chaplain described going to divinity school "unaffiliated," without a particular faith community, and casting about for some kind of group that reflected her own distrust of organized religion and her "belief in the power of belief." She says, "Actually I morph myself so easily and I know that freaks a lot of people out. Like how can you be a humanist and pray to my God and join me in prayer? . . . And it's . . . an honor for me to do that. This is your belief. I have my belief. It's beyond tolerance, because I really believe that that's reality for that person and who am I to say that my reality is more valid or any better?"

This chaplain is an exemplary liberal subject. For her, it matters not to whom you pray—as long as you don't believe your God or your reality is any more real than the next. That is, what has now become truly incommensurable is any religion that claims to know the truth. When I asked the ECM chaplain whether any Pentecostal chaplains were on staff she said, "There are actually very few because most conservative fundamental religious people can't meet the patient where he or she is, so they're not good chaplains. Because they have to proselytize and they have to evangelize. And that's not what chaplaincy is about. Chaplaincy is: if you are a Wiccan I'm going to help you and your coven deal with your illness—especially if it's toward end of life stuff. . . . Will I get you blood from a chicken? I really can't do that. But boy, can I arrange it so that possibly someone can get a day pass home to have a cleansing ritual done by your Haitian shaman? I'd go for that."

The Life Thing

The ECM chaplain believes in belief and thus can accept almost anything a patient believes. But besides the fact that belief has become so emptied of its content, that belief itself is the object of belief, one of the things we can also glean from this chaplain's comments is the "optional" quality of religion in a hospital.[4] That is, despite the fact that medicine and religion have a closely intertwined history and that the hospital initially emerged as a religious institution (Lee 2002), religion is today optional in a way that medicine, as science, is not. Despite, or in some sense because of, JCAHO's measures, the hospital chaplain is a marginal figure, existing on the sidelines of the "real" work done by the medical professionals. Thus the ECM chaplain notes above that she can "help you deal with your illness—*especially if it's toward end of life stuff.*" As Jessica Muller and Barbara Koenig point out, "Once defined as dying, patients are thrust to the periphery of medical work. 'Dying' becomes an exit label symbolizing patients' passages beyond the physicians' professional domain" (1988, 371). Thus the chaplaincy plays a central role in palliative care and is called only in unusual circumstances to the emergency room.

One rabbi I spoke with highlighted the optional character of chaplaincy: "I tell the patients that talking to me is optional, I'm one of the only people in the hospital you don't *have* to talk to. So you get through the physical stuff and if there's any metaphysical stuff you would like to discuss with me, I'm there." But a Roman Catholic priest from Manila put it most plainly. He noted that there is a chaplain assigned to each ward except the emergency room. He explained this by saying, "Especially in the [United] States now, the religion is not considered. In the ER they treat the medical thing . . . which is the *work* . . . the priority in a sense." "[The priority] is the body?" I ask. He replies, "That's why they bring them to the medical room."

In fact, all the chaplains I spoke with articulated a great respect for the work of the doctors, and their attempts to bring the body back to health. To illustrate this, one chaplain told me the story of a family who was struggling with the imminent death of a family member. In the presence of the chaplain they were challenging the cardiologist saying, "Can't we do more?" The cardiologist was saying, "Don't you understand? I'll never know how heart-breaking this is for you, but for me this is, on a totally different level, a terrible failure. I want this to work, this is what I do. I live for taking these people back to health, and it's not working. Of course it doesn't affect me the way that affects you, but in a different way, it's horrible." The chaplain recounting this story commented that "I think he's an exceptional doctor, but he's not that exceptional in the sense that I think all these doctors really want the life thing to work."

To my mind there are several interesting moments in this interaction. For a doctor, the death of his patient is a professional failure. "I live for taking these people back to health, and it's not working." The doctor is making a claim for two tragedies, the tragedy of not being able to make the "life thing" work, to use the chaplain's words, and the tragedy of losing someone you love. He comments, "Of course it doesn't affect me the way it affects you, but in a different way, it's horrible." He is acknowledging that giving up on this particular life means something very different to the doctor and to the patient. What medicine cares about and what the patient cares about differ in significant ways (Good 1998). The priority, in the hospital, is to make the life thing work. When it doesn't, when the life thing has failed, and the patient has exited what Mary-Jo DelVecchio Good calls the biotechnical embrace (Good 2001), there is more room for the chaplaincy.

Walking the Line

But although the chaplains repeatedly expressed their deep respect for the doctors and their work, they did occasionally voice their frustration at the fact that "the life thing" always trumped other concerns. One woman, a Protestant chaplain close to retirement, confided that almost every chaplain had had the experience of a doctor walking into the room and, "starting to talk to the patient when we're standing there talking, and just ignoring us. And if the team comes in, the team will do that too. And some chaplains will say, 'Excuse me, could I have five minutes?' And I know I could do that, and I wouldn't be scared to do that, but I usually say to the patient, 'I'll be back, my schedule is more flexible.' And a lot of times I'll say it loud enough so they can hear it too, and leave."

She explains to me that "in the hospital, the clergy is not the kingpin. It's the surgeons, physicians. [Patients] come to hospitals for *medical healing,* and . . . there's sometimes an invisibility about chaplains" (emphasis added). At such moments, the chaplains begin to talk about the line in the hospital that chaplains cannot cross. And so, for example, when I asked a director of chaplaincy about those moments when the culture of medicine comes into conflict with his religious beliefs, he responded, "We do have to walk a line here, where on the one hand, the one thing that a chaplain will never do is to speak ill of anyone else on the medical team. . . . But the other part of the line is, our main role as a chaplain is to minister to the patient." There is a tension here between attending to the patient and the desire to please the hospital administration. Another chaplain adds, "We aren't allowed to proselytize and preach. We'd be bounced out of a job if we did that."

In an effort to counter this invisibility and to become "legible" to hospital bureaucracies and staff, chaplains have begun to "chart" their visits, writing a summary of their encounter in the patient's medical chart. "It's to make sure the chaplaincy department continues to exist in this hospital," says one chaplain as he dutifully adds his comments to the pages of notes (for a discussion of writing and authority in the hospital, see Good 1994a). The confrontation of the sacred with such bureaucratic forms can be jarring. On rounds with a Catholic chaplain, we visit a man who has just had his prostate removed. In the hall as we wait for the nurses to leave the bedside, the chaplain pulls a glass vial and some cotton wool out of his pants pocket. I am startled by the entry of these objects into the disenchanted space of the hospital corridor, but the chaplain's face is impassive, the act so routine he seems not to realize he's doing it. At the patient's bedside, after a brief introduction and some questions about how the procedure went, the chaplain asks the patient if he would like a prayer for healing and anointing, to which the patient agrees. The chaplain then intones a prayer in a singsong voice and smooths the oil-drenched cotton on his forehead. Afterwards I follow the chaplain to the nurse's station, where he pulls out the patient's chart and attaches a red sticker to the front page. He writes the date, his initials, and the word *anointed* on the sticker. "His passport to heaven," the priest says, deadpan.

The chaplain's joke belies the seriousness of chaplain's writing practices. Chaplains see this practice of writing as essential to ensuring their ongoing presence in the hospital. Through charting, they become more visible to the other hospital staff. As one oncologist recently noted during the Schwartz rounds[5] at Massachusetts General Hospital, "I noticed something recently. The chaplains have been putting notes in the medical chart. I love it. It's been really important to me to see the chaplain putting these notes in because, until a very short time ago, I could never find them. I could never catch up with the chaplains. They were there but they were like phantoms" (Penson et al. 2001, 289).

Existing in the realm of the spirit, phantoms can neither be readily seen nor heard and they are not properly materialized. In the hospital, where the body is the work, not having a body removes the chaplain from the grasp of hospital staff. So although JCAHO's move to make religious care a right seems to sanction the role of religion in the hospital, in fact it moves religion into the material realm. Chaplains need to be materialized. That is, that religion is "on the front sheet" belies the important reality that the modern American hospital is an institution that privileges the healing of the human body through scientific techniques, and that chaplaincy must be understood as some kind of vaguely conceived psycho-social intervention if it is to be acceptable to the ideology of medical care (for a discussion of the professionalization of chaplaincy in the United States, see Vries, Berlinger, and Cadge 2008). Today, writing—as a form of legitimacy—enables the chaplains to be caught, to be brought inside the structure and law of the hospital. No longer either "lone ranger figures" or "phantoms," chaplains have become in part functionaries, issuing passports to heaven.

Yet to leave the story of chaplaincy there, to see chaplains merely as bureaucrats of the sacred would be an oversimplification. Although I think the tendency to subsume religion within the culture concept has had some unfortunate consequences, in particular that it leads to a psychologized notion of spirituality that ignores the specificity of particular religious beliefs and practices, still I recognize the multiple and conflicting discourses through which chaplains operate. As one chaplain put it, "It's about finding a language that will get you in the door." Her comment highlights the negotiation of multiple and conflicting discourses—there's how you frame your work to hospital administration, there's what you write on charts, and then there's what you actually say and do with patients (compare Vries, Berlinger, and Cadge 2008).

As an anthropologist listening to the chaplains, I began to see them as playing a very specific role in the hospital. In some sense they were there to provide another way of listening—*une autre écoute*—in Stefania Pandolfo's terms (2006). In a setting where what is most often being listened for is the symptom, this kind of listening is a radical departure, and gestures to something beyond just the material, beyond the body-as-diseased, beyond death as failure, to something potentially more powerful than medicine (for a discussion of chaplaincy and metamorphosis, see Vries, Berlinger, and Cadge 2008, 23–24).[6]

Several of the chaplains I interviewed said they chose to work in the hospital setting because it was there, in the midst of suffering, that they felt the really important theological questions were being raised. One of the full-time Protestant chaplains described having had a part-time summer job at a Boston-area hospital: "I was quite taken with the academic medical center, that there was so much happening here, and a lot of it was people were questioning the meaning of their life—and where was God—very vividly." She contrasted this with the church setting where people are not always "on the edge, not in crisis, or hanging on by their fingernails."

In this vein, one chaplain talked about the fact that although she was very well trained by the neurology team in the hospital to accept the definition of brain death, still she has "seen some things" that make you question what's going on. "I have seen some things, I think that there . . . sometimes there's been dire predictions from the medical team, and everybody buys into it, then the person walks out the door! . . . I love stuff like that. I love it, because it reminds me that one of the greatest hospitals in the world isn't always right on the money. That there is something besides the intellectual, medical approach."

Another chaplain tells me how hard it is when patients ask him to pray for a miracle after the doctor says there is nothing more that can be done. "When the doctor says that's it, I believe them. I think maybe the miracle is for acceptance." I push him on this, asking him if he thinks that prayer can change medical outcomes. "Yes I do," he says, and smiles at his inconsistency. He tells me then about a doctor who has a sign on his wall that says, "If the patient gets better it doesn't mean you got the diagnosis right." There is always, the chaplain says, the possibility for things we don't understand.

The chaplains, at the very minimum, consistently listen for things we don't understand, or things that don't fit the medical narrative. One chaplain reflected on a situation in which "it really bothered me that I had all this information from the medical establishment. How do I shut that out and hear her story for the first time? So that's actually my dream role, that I don't read the patient's chart. I go in, I hear their story. I find out how it's affected their life. How they see themselves as spiritual or psychosocial beings. You know, what does that mean? Do they find meaning in this? That's huge."

It's important to notice, as I mentioned, that this other way of listening is not equally valued throughout the hospital. On the one hand, the chaplains are welcomed onto the palliative care team. On the other, the one area of the hospital that has no assigned chaplain is the emergency ward. In palliative care, the "life thing" has not worked, and medicine can afford to allow dying patients recourse to other means: a Haitian patient is given a pass to participate in a voodoo ritual, a young woman is allowed to spend her last day out of doors. But in the emergency room, the life of the body is at stake and chaplains are called in only when a person's "belief" seems to be getting in the way of medical recovery.

But perhaps this other listening is most difficult to sustain on the psychiatric wards where religion and particular demons and deities often emerge in the patient's delusions. "Hearing God's voice," said one psychiatric nurse, "that's always something that we worry about." In the psychiatric ward, the symptom is often articulated in religious terms or spiritual terms, precisely the terms through which the chaplains have learned to listen differently. If a patient's spirituality is a symptom of disease how can the chaplain do her work? A protestant chaplain says, "Often in the psych ward, the psychosis has people saying that they're Jesus Christ, and the psychiatrists are often wary of spirituality in that setting. . . . If the patient is not in the real world either for brain injury or mental illness, I can pray with them but I can't be present to them in the same ways."

A Muslim chaplain described meeting a man on the locked ward. When he entered the room, the patient stood up. The chaplain introduced himself by saying, "I am imam." But the patient responded, "I am the caliph." For the chaplain this meant that the patient saw himself as a reformer of the religion, a bishop, someone an imam would have to defer to. "So I couldn't help, I stood with him and talked with him." "So what did you do?" I ask. "I just run away! [laughs] I couldn't do nothing. I told him, 'Are you sure?' And he said, 'Oh yes. I'm this [the caliph].' And his eyes were so serious in a way that I was afraid to disagree with him. He was looking at me as if sparks could come from them, so I was afraid of looking at him or telling him anything."

One Protestant chaplain in particular reflected at length at the experience of being a religious figure on the psychiatric ward. She noted that it's a "fascinating area because it's really a place where the medical culture and the culture of religiosity can clash." She continued, "I think, the way I understand it right at the moment, the religiosity of patients . . . makes clinicians quite suspicious, and is quickly put into the box of psychosis, which many, many, many times makes absolute sense to me." But there was a kind of uneasiness to this chaplain's speech, and she went on to describe a category of patients where the diagnosis didn't always make "absolute sense." She described patients who were "surprisingly religious all of a sudden, and they may not have been religious before they came to the hospital, but now they are, and is this a part of their psychiatric illness? Or is it a part of—well, in religious terms we would say—a conversion experience?"

She tells me about one such case in detail—a woman who had been asking for books on Buddhism and Christianity. The chaplain gave her a book and the next day went back to visit her on the ward. She explains:

> And then the next day I came up to the unit again, and she was sobbing in the community room and telling me how she [had been] having this powerful, creative, religious force and energy that she was working at shaping within herself and how she could connect with God, and that then made her so happy, and so energetic, and so whatnot. And now she took the medication and it actually started working, and her religiosity was gone, and she just experienced the loss of her connection to God as she had experienced it before, and was just—

Upon my remarking that this loss was a tragedy, she continued:

> It was a tragedy for her! Now, for me then, I was sitting there—and of course she was trying to pull me into, "Don't you agree chaplain? These psychiatrists are no good!"—and all I knew ... to do was to say to myself, "She experienced a loss, and I know how to stay with loss, and sort of support someone in that."

The chaplain paused for a moment and then continued speaking. "But it kind of got to me when she leaned over and she said, 'Well, what would you feel if they would give you a pill and you couldn't pray any-more?' And I thought, 'Gee, well.'"

So, although it is difficult and not always possible to find another way of listening to psychotic patients, I think this case presents a moment of rupture, when the chaplain is not simply reframing what the patient says into familiar—often medical or psychological—terms. Instead the chaplain's own world is momentarily put into question, her status as the one with the sanity and the proper ways of proceeding, troubled: "Gee, well." *What if they gave me a pill and I couldn't pray anymore?* Part of what this chapter is asking is what it means to listen differently, to learn something we didn't already know, to be genuinely confronted and disturbed by our own or other ways of doing things. What would it mean to be less quick to make all cultural and religious practice equivalent, to hold open the possibility, ultimately, that we too, as liberal subjects, may be converted?

An openness to conversion, in the sense I intend it here, allows for the possibility that the self will be transformed in the process of translation. Translation, when conversion is at stake, is not about "assimilating [the other] into a pre-existing discourse or configuration of the self. It requires an openness to alterity, a radical discontinuity of experience" (Pandolfo 2007, 332). This openness entails a risk, the risk that the self will not be the same after engaging in the (radical) act of translation. It means that translation is neither fully possible nor impossible, but rather is an act that can reconstitute the self and its ways of thinking and acting in the world. As chaplains, doctors, nurses, administrators, researchers—as liberal subjects—our challenge is to avoid simply reinscribing the other as yet another version of the self. By practicing a form of listening described by the chaplain in the psychiatric ward, in which what is at stake is our most deeply held convictions, our ways of living in the world, translation again becomes a radical act.

Notes

1. For a discussion of the way power influences the direction of translation, see Asad 1993a; for a discussion of the way migrants to Italy translate their experiences into narratives that the state can assimilate, see Giordano (2008).
2. For Foucault this meant turning one's own body and one's life into a work of art. In the piece, a jointly edited interview, "On the Genealogy of Ethics: An Overview of Work in Progress," he wrote, "From the idea that the self is not given to us, I think that there is only one practical consequence: we have to create ourselves as a work of art (1997, 262).
3. For a discussion of sincerity in Protestant prayer, see Keane (2002).
4. As Talal Asad puts it, "Religion is indeed now optional in a way that science is not. Scientific practices, techniques, knowledges, permeate and create the very fibers of social life in ways that religion no longer does. In that sense, religion today *is* a perspective (or an 'attitude,' as Geertz sometimes calls it), but science is not" (1993b, 49).
5. The Schwartz rounds at the Massachusetts General are "a monthly multi-disciplinary forum where caregivers reflect on important psychosocial issues faced by patients, their families, and their caregivers, and gain insight and support from fellow staff members" (Penson et al. 2001, 286).
6. As will become apparent, I am interested not just in the metamorphosis of the patient but also the chaplain.

References

Asad, Talal. 1993a. "The Concept of Cultural Translation in British Social Anthropology." In *Genealogies of Religion: Discipline and Reasons of Power in Christianity and Islam*. Baltimore, Md.: Johns Hopkins University Press.

———. 1993b. "The Construction of Religion as an Anthropological Category." In *Genealogies of Religion: Discipline and Reasons of Power in Christianity and Islam*. Baltimore, Md.: Johns Hopkins University Press.

———. 2007. *On Suicide Bombing*. New York: Columbia University Press.

Cadge, Wendy, Jeremy Freese, and Nicholas A. Christakis. 2008. "The Provision of Hospital Chaplaincy in the United States: A National Overview." *Southern Medical Journal* 101(6): 626–30. doi 10.1097/SMJ.0b013e3181706856.

Foucault, Michel. 1997. "On the Genealogy of Ethics: An Overview of Work in Progress." In *Ethics: Subjectivity and Truth*, edited by Paul Rabinow. New York: New Press.

Giordano, Cristiana. 2008. "Practices of Translation and the Making of Migrant Subjectivities in Contemporary Italy." *American Ethnologist* 35(4): 588–606.

Good, Byron J. 1994a. "How Medicine Constructs Its Objects." In *Medicine, Rationality, and Experience: An Anthropological Perspective* (Lewis Henry Morgan Lectures). Cambridge: Cambridge University Press.

———. 1994b. "Medical Anthropology and the Problem of Belief." In *Medicine, Rationality, and Experience: An Anthropological Perspective* (Lewis Henry Morgan lectures). Cambridge: Cambridge University Press.

Good, Mary-Jo DelVecchio. 1998. *American Medicine: The Quest for Competence.* Berkeley: University of California Press.

———. 2001. "The Biotechnical Embrace." *Culture, Medicine and Psychiatry* 25(4): 395–410.

Hage, Ghassan. 2003. "'Comes a Time We Are All Enthusiasm': Understanding Palestinian Suicide Bombers in Times of Exighophobia." *Public Culture* 15(1): 65–89.

Hahn, Robert A., and Arthur Kleinman. 1983. "Belief as Pathogen, Belief as Medicine: 'Voodoo Death' and the 'Placebo Phenomenon' in Anthropological Perspective." *Medical Anthropology Quarterly* 4(4): 16–19.

Keane, Webb. 2002. "Sincerity, 'Modernity,' and the Protestants." *Cultural Anthropology* 17(1): 65–92.

Kleinman, Arthur, and Peter Benson. 2006. "Anthropology in the Clinic: The Problem of Cultural Competency and How to Fix It." *PLoS Medicine.* 3(10): 1673–76.

Lee, Simon J. Craddock. 2002. "In a Secular Spirit: Strategies of Clinical Pastoral Education." *Health Care Analysis* 10: 339–56.

Muller, Jessica H., and Barbara Koenig. 1988. "On the Boundary of Life and Death: The Definition of Dying by Medical Residents." In *Biomedicine Examined: Culture, Illness, and Healing,* edited by Margaret Lock and Deborah Gordon. Dordrecht, Neth.: Kluwer Academic Publishers.

Murray, Stuart J. 2006. "Thanatopolitics: On the Use of Death for Mobilizing Political Life." *Polygraph* 18: 191–215.

Pandolfo, Stefania. 2006. "'B"Ìt N"Anni Hnaya'" (Je Veux Chanter Ici) Voix et Témoignage en Marge D'une Rencontre Psychiatrique." *Arabica* LIII(2): 232–80.

———. 2007. "'The Burning': Finitude and the Politico-Theological Imagination of Illegal Migration." *Anthropological Theory* 7(3): 329–63.

Penson, Richard T., Rushdia Z. Yusuf, Bruce A. Chabner, Joanne P. Lafrancesca, Michael McElhinny, Albert S. Axelrad, and Thomas J. Lynch Jr. 2001. "Losing God." *The Oncologist* 6(3): 286–97.

Povinelli, Elizabeth A. 2001. "Radical Worlds: The Anthropology of Incommensurability and Inconceivability." *Annual Review of Anthropology* 30: 319–34.

Vries, Raymond de, Nancy Berlinger, and Wendy Cadge. 2008. "Lost in Translation: The Chaplain's Role in Health Care." *Hastings Center Report* 38(6): 23–27.

Weber, Max. 1948. *Max Weber: Essays in Sociology,* edited and translated by H. H. Gerth and C. Wright Mills. London: Routledge and Kegan Paul.

Young, Allan. 1996. "Suffering and the Origins of Traumatic Memory." *Daedalus* 125(1): 245–260.

Chapter 5

Clinician-Patient Matching

SARAH S. WILLEN

THE PROSPECT of "matching" patients with providers on the basis of shared language, race-ethnicity, or cultural background has recently emerged as a potentially promising strategy for reducing disparities in mental health outcomes. Despite considerable interest in matching over the past fifteen years, especially in psychology, it remains unclear whether these efforts are meaningful, mythical, or perhaps even misguided. Although a wide variety of studies have been conducted in recent years to assess matching's efficacy, findings remain equivocal. In the early 1990s, a number of large-scale quantitative studies demonstrated positive associations between concordant patient-provider matches and a variety of standard outcome measures (Snowden, Hu, and Jerrell 1995; Sue et al. 1991). Yet the bulk of subsequent research has demonstrated either a much weaker relationship between matching and improved outcomes than previously hypothesized or no relationship at all (Maramba and Hall 2002; Shin et al. 2005). These quantitative studies, however, involve multiple limitations. First, it is often unclear how basic concepts—among them concepts of culture, ethnicity, and matching—are operationalized for research purposes. Second, they offer little insight into how matching is conceptualized, practiced, or rejected as a therapeutic strategy in everyday clinical settings.

This chapter draws on qualitative interviews conducted with psychiatrists, psychologists, and social workers to cast a revealing, critical light on the controversial and complicated issue of clinician-patient matching. Clinicians interviewed represent a wide array of clinical settings, including academic medical centers' inpatient and outpatient clinics, private and community hospital inpatient and outpatient services, and community health centers. Our findings suggest that matching, which is not employed systematically among the clinicians interviewed, is regarded with considerable ambivalence. Ideal typical notions of a match are difficult to conceptualize and even more difficult to implement. Moreover, clinicians note that the very idea of matching may be based on problematic common-sense assumptions about processes of cultural or racial-ethnic identification; about the optimal relationship between patient and care provider; or about the factors most likely to facilitate patient-provider rapport and meaningful therapeutic alliances. Overall, clinicians' comments raise challenging questions about the viability of matching as a strategy for remediating differences in mental health outcomes among more and less vulnerable patient populations.

Clinician-Patient Matching: Definitions and Motives

The term clinician-patient matching (or doctor-patient matching) is used to describe efforts to pair patients with care providers on the basis of shared language competence, shared cultural or racial-ethnic background (generally in keeping with the U.S. racial-ethnic pentad), or a combination of the two. These forms of matching are driven by a variety of sometimes overlapping motives: instrumental, diagnostic, therapeutic, and economic (see table 5.1). In this discussion, I concentrate on the first three sets.

Table 5.1   Motives for Clinician-Patient Matching

Motive	Goal
Instrumental	To facilitate direct communication between care provider and patient without the need for a translator or interpreter
Diagnostic	To ensure maximal clinician sensitivity to - culturally influenced configurations of symptoms - culturally influenced idioms of distress - the relationship between distress and patient's broader lifeworld context To yield "better" or more accurate diagnoses
Therapeutic	To maximize utilization rates of available services To prevent treatment drop-out To lengthen duration of treatment To achieve greater rapport and stronger therapeutic alliance To achieve greater patient satisfaction To improve treatment outcomes
Economic	To decrease use of expensive services (such as emergency care, inpatient care) in favor of lower-cost outpatient clinical services

Source: Author's compilation.

Although the two primary forms of matching—language-based and cultural or racial-ethnic—are often elided in practice, they are substantively different.[1] Language matching, or the pairing of patients and providers on the basis of shared language competence, is meant to facilitate direct communication. Such communication is generally regarded as preferable to triadic clinical interactions involving a translator or interpreter, whose presence is generally assumed to influence both the content and the dynamics of clinical interactions (chapter 3, this volume). The primary aim of language matching, which can have important consequences for diagnosis and treatment, is instrumental; it is best understood as a technical fix designed to resolve a technical problem. Understood this way, language matching does not depend on any inherent or intrinsic features of either the patient or the provider. For instance, a Mexican American patient who speaks Spanish as a first language might be regarded as an appropriate match with a care provider of Irish American heritage for whom Spanish is an acquired second language.

Cultural or racial-ethnic matching, by contrast, aims to resolve more subtle issues that have been hypothesized to influence diagnosis and treatment, including, in particular, matters of mutual intelligibility and interpersonal dynamics. In contrast with language matching, this second form of matching hinges on the intrinsic characteristics of both patient and provider. In diagnostic terms, cultural or racial-ethnic matching is promoted as a way to maximize clinician sensitivity to culturally influenced configurations of symptoms or idioms of distress. It may also be promoted as a way to ensure maximum clinician sensitivity to the relationship between patients' distress and their broader lifeworld contexts. Ultimately, this form of matching has been touted as a way to achieve better or more accurate diagnoses. In therapeutic terms, matching has been posited as a way to achieve higher utilization rates among particular patient populations, to reduce rates of treatment dropout and increase duration of treatment, to strengthen rapport or therapeutic alliance, to achieve greater patient satisfaction from treatment, and ultimately to improve treatment outcomes. A fourth motive for matching also merits mention: the possibility that matching might reduce overall costs by reducing utilization rates of more expensive emergency and inpatient mental health services (Jerrell 1995).

Literature on Matching: Initial Enthusiasm, Waning Support

The concept of matching is the product of a changing—and increasingly hyperdiverse—American sociopolitical climate in which mental health researchers began paying attention to how processes of social classification and categorization can affect the mental health status of nonmainstream and, to a lesser extent, mainstream groups (Sue 2003). Research revealing disparities in patterns of mental health care utilization and outcomes contributed to the emergence of a movement in favor of more culturally competent care, or therapeutic approaches driven in part by "the belief that people should not only appreciate and recognize other cultural groups but also be able to effectively work with them" (Sue 2003, 440). In this sociopolitically dynamic context, matching has been put forth as one among other possible strategies for achieving this hard-to-define objective (Banks 1999; Maramba and Hall 2002; Sue 1998).

Early enthusiasm for matching relied on evidence that patients appeared to prefer providers of similar cultural or racial-ethnic backgrounds (Atkinson and Lowe 1995; Atkinson et al. 1989; Coleman, Wampold, and Casali 1995; Constantine 2002; Proctor and Rosen 1981; Terrell and Terrell 1984; Watkins and Terrell 1988; Watkins et al. 1989), and that racially or ethnically matched clinicians had greater credibility with their patients, at least in the initial states of treatment (Sue and Zane 1987). Support for matching also relied on evidence that "mismatches" can introduce misunderstandings, miscommunication, and cultural biases into clinical interactions. As Sung-Man Shin and colleagues (2005) explain, such forms of miscommunication have been held responsible, at least in part, for underuse of mental health services, higher rates of treatment dropout, and poorer outcomes for minority patients (Erdur, Rude, and Baron 2003; Flaskerud and Liu 1991; Sue 1998; Sue et al. 1991). Early studies suggested that matched patients tended to remain in treatment longer (Sue 1998; Sue et al. 1991), be higher-functioning at the conclusion of therapy (Sue 1998; Sue et al. 1991), and use fewer emergency services than unmatched patients (Snowden, Hu, and Jerrell 1995).

Despite the enthusiasm generated by these preliminary findings, more recent research—consisting primarily of quantitative studies published in psychology journals—has provided little evidence in favor of matching. These findings remain consistent across analogue studies, which measure preferences for matched versus unmatched care providers (see Atkinson 1985; Atkinson, Furlong, and Poston 1986; Atkinson and Lowe 1995; Bennett and BigFoot-Sipes 1991); archival studies, which assess the impact of matching on a variety of outcome measures (see Flaskerud and Liu 1991; Fujino, Okazaki, and Young 1994; Mathews et al. 2002; Sue et al. 1991); and process-outcome studies (see Erdur, Rude, and Baron 2003; Jones 1978, 1982; Ricker, Nystul, and Waldo 1999). Current research suggests that matching appears to have no significant impact, among other factors, on duration of treatment, therapeutic alliance, overall functioning (Maramba and Hall 2002; Shin et al. 2005; Takeuchi, Sue, and Yeh 1995), or treatment outcome (Erdur, Rude, and Baron 2003; Fujino, Okazaki, and Young 1994; Jones 1978, 1982; Maramba and Hall 2002; Rosenheck and Seibyl 1998; Sue et al. 1991).

Despite the strength and consistency of these findings, the assumption that matching is inherently beneficial seems to have become normalized "to the point at which such matching is commonplace in psychotherapy and case management services today" (Karlsson 2005, 114, citing Mathews et al. 2002). This curious contradiction—between widespread, even common-sense support for matching, on one hand, and lack of evidence in its favor, on the other—makes it particularly important to explore how matching is conceptualized and applied in real-life clinical settings. To date, very few studies have taken up this challenge (but see Chang and Berk 2009; Liggan, Liggan, and Kay 1999). Before reporting our findings, it is helpful to consider several problems with the logic that has put matching forward as a disparity-reduction strategy worth pursuing.

Clinician-Patient Matching: Critical Perspectives

Research on matching has been criticized on political as well as method-ological and epistemological grounds. Methodological problems include the lack of prospective studies, that is, clinical trials designed in accor-dance with the demands of evidence-based medicine;[2] the paucity of research in actual psychotherapy settings; and inattention to therapist variables such as "cultural sensitivity" (Karlsson 2005).

A fourth methodological problem stems from the lack of clear or consis-tent operational definitions of either race-ethnicity or culture, particularly within contemporary environments of hyperdiversity. How are patients' cultural or racial-ethnic background identified, and by whom? Do provi-ders make such determinations? Do patients? How are individuals who identify themselves as having mixed heritage classified? How are matches identified and defined by researchers? Whether identifications are made on the basis of self-report, ascribed classification, or some combination of the two, the lack of methodological clarity in the studies cited makes it dif-ficult to establish what, in specific, is being matched or measured in any given study. Additional categorical ambiguity is further introduced by the fact that race-ethnicity and culture are often used interchangeably.

These largely neglected methodological problems, however, merely scratch the surface of a much deeper epistemological problem. However defined, clinician-patient matches typically rely on reified forms of catego-rization and classification based on the United States racial-ethnic pentad, a widely employed classificatory model that specifies just five categories: white, black, Asian, Pacific Islander, and American Indian–Alaskan Native. A sixth classifier, Hispanic/Latino, is defined as a cross-cutting cat-egory that may apply to individuals within several racial-ethnic categories (generally white or black). There is nothing obvious or intuitive about this particular classificatory scheme; to the contrary, it reflects a complicated history of labeling, discrimination, and exclusion in the United States. Furthermore, ascriptions of these categories do not necessarily correlate with individuals' self-descriptions. Nonetheless, it has consistently been used to investigate the clinical implications of clinician-patient matching and other forms of "culturally competent" care (for a variation on this scheme, see Sue et al. 1991; Takeuchi, Sue, and Yeh 1995).

From an anthropological perspective, eliding race-ethnicity and culture considerably distorts the complexity of social reality. A vast body of literature has examined how systems of classification mask such complexity, especially when recruited in support of explicit or implicit political agendas (for example, Bowker and Star 1999; Brodkin 1998; Ngai 2004; Waters 1999). If the category white includes Americans of western and eastern Europe, South America, and Middle East origin; black includes African Americans, Caribbean Americans, and African immigrants; and Asian lumps together individuals of Indian, Chinese, Japanese, Korean, and Filipino descent, then how useful can these terms be in clinical practice? Given the social constructedness of race-ethnicity, the reductive nature of the pentad, and the silence about matching techniques in the literature, it is not difficult to accept Roger Karlsson's assertion that research on matching has been plagued by "an abundance of uncontrolled within-group variables" and "difficulties in forming ethnically homogeneous groups for comparisons" (2005, 113).

Findings: Key Themes

The semi-structured, one-on-one interviews our group conducted with clinicians included an open-ended question designed to elicit their perspectives on the issue of clinician-patient matching. Interviews, which were transcribed and coded using the Atlas.ti software program, shed considerable light on the challenges and dilemmas associated with matching as a potential strategy for coping with hyperdiversity. Key themes that arose, and that are explored shortly, include language issues; tensions between the particularity of the matching model and the universality of professional paradigms; competing characterizations of matching as either meaningful, mythical, or misguided; psychodynamic considerations; resistance to matching; and institutional considerations. I consider each of these themes in turn.

The Inseparability of Linguistic and Cultural Concerns

Clinicians identified the technical challenge posed by lack of shared language as particularly problematic. Many spoke about the degree to which sharing a language of communication—either directly or, when necessary, through an interpreter—is fundamental to adequate mental health care.

In one particularly memorable case, a psychiatrist described a Chinese cancer patient who, because he spoke no English, was mistakenly identified as mentally ill, placed in a seclusion room, and chemically sedated after a particularly galling moment of linguistic incomprehensibility. The reason for the patient's precipitating outburst, subsequent misdiagnosis, and improper sedation became clear only when an interpreter fluent in Cantonese was brought in to help facilitate a psychiatric consult.

Most clinicians seemed resigned to the fact that their clinical teams do not include mental health care providers fluent in all of their patients' native languages. In light of this enduring constraint, many affirmed the role played by interpreters on clinical teams (compare chapter 3, this volume). One psychologist employed at an in-patient psychiatric ward explained that her hospital's interpreter service "has always been really helpful." When asked whether having a third person present in clinical interactions might be a barrier to establishing rapport, the psychologist explained it this way:

> Well, I think it could be. But . . . most of the people here, in my experience, they—not everyone, but a lot of them—are actually pretty good. . . . for the most part, I don't feel . . . they get in the way. In fact, it's not uncommon for an interpreter to talk to a patient, and the patient will turn to speak to the interpreter, and the interpreter will tell us, "I'm gonna tell the patient to continue talking to you guys, and I'll just talk to her, or talk to him, from the side. So that she can see your facial expressions, and you can see hers."

At the same time, some clinicians—especially those who are fluent in multiple languages—explained that interpreter-mediated clinical interactions will always be less than ideal. A mental health counselor employed on a culturally specific mental health unit noted that "you lose so much" because some patients "don't feel comfortable having a translator. Or they don't feel [they are] relating or even making a bond with the provider, so they don't feel that they're understood." Overall, clinicians' comments suggest that some regard direct, unmediated communication as a fundamental requirement for satisfactory mental health care. For others, especially those who work regularly with a multilingual patient population, competent translation or interpretation services are considered sufficient.

Another important issue involved the differential impact of language differences within different types of clinical interactions. As one psychologist noted, "I think it really depends if it's going to be your psychiatrist who's doing medication management, or a therapist."

For these clinicians, possibilities for matching were variously interpreted in terms of patient's primary language, racial-ethnic background (typically in accordance with the pentad), or cultural background—elements that are often difficult, or even impossible, to separate. Because language and culture are so deeply intertwined, it is certainly possible that basic linguistic comprehensibility can exist without mutual understanding of the nuances of patient experience. This challenge can arise in interactions between native and non-native speakers of any given language (English, Spanish, Mandarin, and so on) or in interactions between native speakers of a given language whose cultures are nonetheless substantially different (that is, Argentine versus Puerto Rican Spanish speakers, French versus Congolese French speakers, Lebanese versus Egyptian Arabic speakers, and so on).

Tension Between the Particularism of the Matching Model and the Universalism of Professional Paradigms

A second key theme involved what some clinicians perceived as an inherent conflict between the particularist logic of the matching model and the universalism of their professional models of clinical care. Professional models of psychiatry, psychology, and social work tend to be grounded in universalizing assumptions about the nature of the human mind, brain, and psyche; about the skills required to be a competent clinician; or both. For some critics, the fundamental problem with matching is its presumption that shared personal experience is necessary for treatment to be adequate or sufficient. According to one psychiatrist at a major medical center,

> you don't have to have that same kind of experience as that patient, you just have to be aware of what the variables are. The only time I would say that emphatically that statement is true [is] if you're talking about a language barrier. . . . But if communication is not an issue, I don't think that matching per se means that there's superior care. . . . Because then you're saying that because the physician has . . . to be familiar with all the things that the patient is going through in order to deliver superior care. I don't think that's true.

This psychiatrist contends that good psychiatric care hinges on clinicians' attentiveness to key variables that may affect patients' experience. This almost mathematical emphasis on variables that can be isolated—as opposed to dynamics that might be probed or understood in hermeneutic depth—seems consistent with contemporary psychiatry's universalizing tendencies.

Matching As Meaningful

Although some clinicians were adamantly opposed to the idea of racial-ethnic or cultural matching, the majority regarded it as a potentially advantageous technique for establishing rapport or cultivating a therapeutic alliance. For one psychologist, "I think that to the best of our ability to get people from similar, the same or similar, cultural background is a huge advantage." Another psychologist agreed:

> Personally through my own experiences, I've come to believe that the ideal is cultural matching. . . . There's a lot of evidence . . . that the best predictor of response to psychotherapy is therapeutic alliance. Best predictor of therapeutic alliance is perceived similarity. . . . There's no question that people who are from the same culture perceive themselves as more similar. And I think it's always an asset to treatment.

In addition to the presumed impact of shared or similar experience on patients' subjective sense of therapeutic alliance, this psychologist's comment also calls attention to a crucial—yet often silent—issue for clinicians: the unspoken assumption that they are capable of providing excellent care to any and all patients. Midway through her explanation of how cultural matching is always an asset to treatment, the psychologist remarked, "Maybe we would all wish that not to be true. Certainly, you know, I would like to—I'm narcissistic myself. I would like to think that I'm the best treatment provider for everyone." As this psychologist notes, a clinician's assumption that she is equally capable of providing optimal care to all patients can create a blind spot which, in certain cases, might obstruct the cultivation of therapeutic rapport between patients and clinicians of different backgrounds.

A psychologist in training on an inpatient ward echoed the view that shared background is likely to increase a patient's level of comfort and a clinician's level of insight. At the same time, she raised two concerns. First, empathy is always required for the development of rapport regardless of any apparent similarity or dissimilarity between patient and provider. Second, a clinician can compensate for the absence of a match by working harder to gain insight into a patient's condition and thus gain the patient's trust. For this psychologist, matching

> has a certain point, because someone who's of the same culture and gender and background—it might be easier to feel comfortable with them . . . and . . . it's probably easier for the patient to feel comfortable with the provider and the provider will probably have more insights into the patient's life, but . . . on the other hand, no two people have exactly the same experience whether they are from the same culture or not, so there's always going to be some sort of need for an empathy from the provider to the patient. So . . . I think it's possible for people from different backgrounds to provide good services, culturally competent services. But I think it probably takes more effort.

Another psychologist contended that racial-ethnic or cultural similarity between patient and provider "just lines up one of the ducks. It doesn't guarantee anything. It just makes it more likely. If you've got someone with the right language, the matching language requirement, who has an interest in working with a population, that's probably the most important."

For these clinicians, shared cultural or racial-ethnic background may confer some benefit in terms of the development of rapport between patients and providers, yet these forms of similarity are but one piece—and a variable piece at best—within a much more complex puzzle.

Matching As Mythical

Whereas some clinicians viewed racial-ethnic or cultural matching as a particularist strategy that contradicts the universalist aims of Western clinical mental health professions, others expressed either reluctance or opposition on other grounds. A number of psychologists intimated that the very idea of matching is illusory, or mythical. Some spoke about the multidimensional nature of human identity and the impossibility of matching along all dimensions. Others noted that matching according to shared characteristics other than culture or race-ethnicity—for instance, gender or sexual orientation—may have a much greater impact on clinician-patient rapport than culturally or racial-ethnically based matching. A psychologist who works with adolescents, for example, explained that "teenage boys tend to want male therapists." Another psychologist, who sometimes does and sometimes does not disclose her own gay identity to her patients, said she has received "a lot of referrals as a lesbian therapist from people who want to see someone who is gay. . . . Maybe it's a matter of what's going to get the person through the door and there are clinicians who are going to be that person, to be that match. . . . It may be very alliance-building, and . . . you may really need that as collateral in beginning your work."

This psychologist raises an important issue concerning the rationale for matching in the first instance. Like "lining up one of the ducks," this clinician suggests particular kinds of perceived similarity may be important for particular patients at the initial stages of entering therapy. For other patients, or for the same patients at other times, perceived similarity may matter less, or not at all.

Given the complex constellation of factors that can influence clinician-patient rapport, these insights raise the question of whether cultural or racial-ethnic matching is possible or, as the following psychologist suggests, utopian or mythical:

> I think that [matching] might work in most situations, but I'm afraid we cannot fragment things as much as we want to. It's impossible; it's utopic. . . . Sometimes there are things that promote a good match that go totally beyond issues of nationality or language or things of that sort. That there is something about the way we are as human beings that is unpredictable.

Put differently, even if it were possible to pin down meaningful definitions of membership within particular cultural or racial-ethnic groups—an effort that entails inherent difficulties—it is not at all clear that matches based on either culture or race-ethnicity would necessarily generate stronger therapeutic alliances than those based on gender, sexual orientation, age, religion, or other factors. Here lies one of the central, and most challenging, clinical implications of hyperdiversity.

Matching As Misguided

Some clinicians implied or explicitly suggested that matching is not just mythical or utopian, but misguided. The clearest illustration was offered by a male social worker who described himself as a Yankee. For him,

> I see everybody, I see people who say, "by the way, I need to see a woman." Or . . . "I'd prefer if I saw a black therapist." Or "I'd prefer . . ." and we end up connecting. It's been rare, really rare where somebody says no way. . . . And I think if they . . . think matching is important . . . the implication is "That's the person who's going to understand me," and while that may be true there is no indication that that's a given. *A woodsman walks into the forest with a long handled axe, and the trees say, Oh good! The handle's made of wood! It must be one of us!* [emphasis added]

For this social worker, similarities in background that appear to signify shared experience and the possibility of stronger rapport may actually hide the seeds of potentially negative or even, if we take his metaphor seriously, destructive consequences.

The Psychodynamics of Matching

The complex therapeutic implications of cultural or racial-ethnic similarity and difference arose most frequently in interviews with psychodynamically inclined clinicians attuned to issues of transference and counter-transference. These clinicians noted that forms of racial-ethnic or cultural difference may signal to patients a normative mainstream to which they hope or wish to belong, a normalizing and oppressive cultural force, or simply an alternative worldview that differs from but may enhance understanding of their own. Some psychologists spoke supportively about certain patients' desires to seek out therapists who feel different:

> The patients I've seen in therapy were English-speaking, of different cultural backgrounds, and it was interesting in our work together to explore that a little bit more, in terms of . . . this person feeling like they needed to fall into this idealized American society, and now their therapist is this

kind of idealized blond-haired, blue-eyed person, and how that might actually affect the relationship, change the relationship, or how that might help the relationship by giving a different perspective that I might be able to offer.

Whereas some patients actively seek out care providers they perceive to be similar to them, others pursue the opposite strategy. A psychiatrist explained it this way:

> Some people have expressed that they don't want to be treated by someone from the same culture. For instance, Dr. M. is from India. There have been patients who come here who say they don't want to see Dr. M. And interestingly, some of them have been from her own culture . . . and . . . there's a wonderful therapist . . . who's African American. On two occasions I've referred patients to her, who come back and say, "I don't want to see her." And they were African American women. One of the women said to me, it was really interesting what she said. It was along the lines of, "You only sent me to her because she's black and I'm black." And it really got into her own negative feelings about herself. . . . And she didn't want—at least this is what the therapist helped me to understand—when she looked at that therapist, [she] saw all the bad stuff she feels about herself as a black person, or just as a person. And she wanted to look at someone . . . who looked more like what she hopes and wants to be, in her mind . . . the same [with] the woman from India, who didn't want to be referred to Dr. M.

Independent of any action on a clinician's part, a patient may project onto his therapist negative feelings about himself, and such projections may interfere with the therapist's effort to cultivate a neutral stance and a relationship of trust and rapport.

Patients may resist culturally or racial-ethnically based matching for other reasons as well. The case of Dr. M., a physician from the remarkably heterogeneous country of India, offers an instructive illustration— as well as a word of caution against resorting too quickly to psychodynamic explanations for avoiding the possibility of a cultural match. From the brief description provided here, we have no way of knowing whether the "Indian" patients the psychiatrist mentioned share Dr. M.'s cultural background, mother tongue, religious affiliation, or caste status. Given the tremendous internal diversity within India as well as the equally substantial diversity among Indian immigrants to the United States, there is reason to be suspicious of any assertion that an "Indian" clinician could be matched unproblematically with an "Indian" patient. Like several South American clinicians interviewed, who indicated that they only "became Latino" in the United States, people of Indian descent may "become Indian" after immigrating to the United States.[3]

Sociocultural Proximity and Resistance to Matching

It is also important to consider how cultural norms, values, beliefs, and practices might shape patients' choice of provider as well as their broader patterns of help-seeking, communicative practices within the context of clinical interactions, and expectations of treatment. For example, if mental health care is stigmatized or sanctioned within one's cultural community, then a patient may be concerned about being negatively judged by a clinician from the same cultural background. A psychologist noted that

> at times where the individual's culture is against psychotherapy or against medication, the patient can come in, and despite the fact that the patient and therapist are from the same culture, actually perceive an extreme difference between themselves and the therapist. Because they begin to feel, well, the therapist is looking at them as weak, or is violating a cultural norm, and they feel very ashamed about that. But on a personal level, I have never once seen that. I have only seen the advantageous side of it.

A patient may also be concerned about the possibility that a clinician from within their community might divulge private and potentially damaging information to other community members. "If the community is small enough," a psychologist indicated, "you don't want someone who you're going to run into repeatedly to know your business."

Institutional Considerations

Three additional matters concerning the application of matching logic in clinical practice merit mention. First, none of our interviewees mentioned any systematic efforts to match patients and providers within their institutions or clinical units. Rather, matching was typically characterized as an informal and occasional practice. (The exception to this rule involved language matching.) Second, lack of diversity among clinical staff was noted as a frequent constraint on the possibility of matching even where it might have been desirable. In many clinical settings, the matching option is simply off the table because there are no available clinicians who share a particular patient's or community's background. In other settings, the pace of everyday practice was described as too fast to worry about issues like matching. A third important issue arose in an interview with a residency training director, who noted that trying to match patients and providers would limit residents' exposure to a diverse patient population. He put forth a strong institutional argument against matching as a clinic-wide strategy, arguing that clinicians in training should instead gain exposure to as broad a patient population as possible.

Conclusion

These qualitative findings raise questions about both the feasibility and the utility of cultural or racial-ethnic matching, especially in mental health care services. Substantial quantitative evidence, including a host of small studies and several large meta-analyses (for example, Maramba and Hall 2002; Shin et al. 2005; Takeuchi, Sue, and Yeh 1995), casts strong doubt on the hypotheses that matching necessarily improves mental health care among minority or immigrant patient populations and that it reduces disparities in outcome. Given the methodological and epistemological limitations of these studies, however, it is difficult to know precisely what they measure.

Not only do the narrative data presented here corroborate these findings, but they also shed light on why certain forms of matching may be less useful than initially postulated. The clinicians interviewed expressed strong support for language matching—that is, an instrumental form of matching based on the extrinsic characteristic of shared linguistic competence—but much less support for cultural or racial-ethnic matching, which is grounded in a sense that shared intrinsic characteristics lead to a stronger therapeutic alliance or to more efficacious treatment.

These findings do not necessarily imply that the majority of clinicians feel competent to negotiate cultural differences in the clinic. In fact, many expressed considerable frustration with the degree to which they feel constrained in their efforts to understand the cultural context of some of their patients' lives. If matching is not an ideal strategy for bridging this gap, then what alternatives merit consideration?

For three decades, medical anthropologists have argued that clinicians ought to amplify their attention to the larger context that shapes patients' experiences of illness, distress, and the clinical relationship (Kleinman 1988; Kleinman, Eisenberg, and Good 1978). In part, this involves attending to the impact of multiple, interlocking processes—social, political, economic, and cultural—on patients' local moral worlds (Kleinman 2006; Kleinman and Benson 2006). It also involves recognizing the difference between cultural difference as a source of disconnect between patients and providers and the role of other factors, including structural differences in social class, education level, level of familiarity with biomedical or hospital settings, level of familiarity or comfort with institutional bureaucracy, or level of scientific literacy (Farmer 2003; Hirsch 2003).

Medical anthropologists also have proposed moving beyond reified and decontextualized notions of culture, especially those animating cultural competence models, to appreciate the role of narrative in organizing biomedical encounters and shaping clinical interactions (Good 1995a, 1995b, 2010; Good and Good 2000). Clinical narratives have powerful social consequences. They affirm relations of power, "emplot" therapeutic trajectories and healing processes (Mattingly 1994), shape the affective dispositions of healers and patients alike (Good et al. 1994) and "direct action and technological interventions" (Good 2010, 276). Indeed, clinical narratives "inscribe treatment experiences on a patient's psyche and soma" (Good 2010, 276). As such, efforts to deliberately co-construct narratives can have a meaningful, positive impact on health care outcomes in mental health and related fields (see, for instance, Kirmayer 2000; Lakes, López, and Garro 2006; Mattingly and Garro 2000).

Certainly what Mattingly describes as clinicians' "chart talk" (1998) and the kind of co-constructed narratives that can emerge in clinical interactions will always differ. As Kimberly Lakes and her colleagues elaborate, however, the key clinical question is not "how much" patients' and clinicians' perspectives should optimally be integrated, but rather whether "the patient and clinician are working from the same shared narrative" (2006, 394). There is reason to believe that careful and deliberate attention to the factors and forces that shape individual patients' experiences—that is, an anthropologically enriched form of good listening, influenced by attention to patients' local moral worlds and to the value of strategic narrative co-construction—will have a more meaningful impact on the health outcomes of patients from nonmainstream cultural backgrounds than more formulaic efforts at racial-ethnic or cultural matching.

Notes

1.   In some cases, "ethnic match" (that is, "matching a client with a therapist of the same ethnicity" [Maramba and Hall 2002, 291]) is distinguished from "cultural match," which is used more generally to suggest a level of cultural competence on the part of the care provider (see, for instance, Maramba and Hall 2002, 294; Sue et al. 1991; Sue and Zane 1987). This manner of distinguishing between the ethnic match (based on shared intrinsic features) and cultural match (based on an extrinsic feature of the provider) is rather confusing, as is the introduction of the more recent notion of "cognitive match" (Zane et al. 2005). Here I use these terms interchangeably to indicate matching on the basis of shared intrinsic features of both patient and provider.

2.   But see Stanley Sue's (2003) comment that the dominance of evidence-based research "is limiting because forms of knowledge based on discovery rather than hypothesis testing are often ignored as important sources of information (967)." This line of critique lends implicit support to our argument that qualitative research methods can yield a diversity of new insights and new information that would not have emerged in a hypothesis-driven quantitative study.

3.   The sociologist Mary Waters (1999) describes an analogous situation among Caribbean immigrants to the United States who "become black" only after settling in their new country of residence and, importantly, who take steps to differentiate themselves from others with similar phenotypic characteristics who are classified in this way.

References

Atkinson, Donald R. 1985. "A Meta-Review of Research on Cross Cultural Counseling and Psychotherapy." *Journal of Multicultural Counseling and Development* 13(4): 138–53.

Atkinson, Donald R., M. J. Furlong, and W. C. Poston. 1986. "Afro-American Preferences for Counselor Characteristics." *Journal of Counseling Psychology* 33(3): 326–30.

Atkinson, Donald R., and S. M. Lowe. 1995. "The Role of Ethnicity, Cultural Knowledge, and Conventional Techniques in Counseling and Psychotherapy." In *Handbook of Multicultural Counseling,* edited by J. G. Ponterotto, J. M. Casas, L. A. Suzuki, and C. M. Alexander. Thousand Oaks, Calif.: Sage Publications.

Atkinson, Donald R., W. Carlos Poston, Michael J. Furlong, and Pauline Mercado. 1989. "Ethnic Group Preferences for Counselor Characteristics." *Journal of Counseling Psychology* 36(1): 68–72.

Banks, Nick. 1999. *White Counselors—Black Clients: Theory, Research and Practice.* Brookfield, Vt.: Ashgate Publishing.

Bennett, Sandra K., and Dolores S. BigFoot-Sipes. 1991. "American Indian and White College Student Preference for Counselor Characteristics." *Journal of Counseling Psychology* 38(4): 440–45.

Bowker, Geoffrey C., and Susan Leigh Star. 1999. *Sorting Things Out: Classification and Its Consequences.* Cambridge, Mass.: MIT Press.

Brodkin, Karen. 1998. *How Jews Became White Folks and What That Says About Race in America.* New Brunswick, N.J.: Rutgers University Press.

Chang, Doris F., and Alexandra Berk. 2009. "Making Cross-Racial Therapy Work: A Phenomenological Study of Clients' Experiences of Cross-Racial Therapy." *Journal of Counseling Psychology* 56(4): 521–36.

Coleman, Hardin L. K., Bruce E. Wampold, and Sherry L. Casali. 1995. "Ethnic Minorities' Rating of Ethnically Similar and European American Counselors: A Meta-Analysis." *Journal of Counseling Psychology* 42(1): 55–64.

Constantine, Madonna G. 2002. "Predictors of Satisfaction with Counseling: Racial and Ethnic Minority Clients' Attitudes Toward Counseling and Ratings of Their Counselor's General and Multicultural Counseling Competence." *Journal of Counseling Psychology* 49(2): 255–63.

Erdur, Ozgur, Stephanie S. Rude, and Augustine Baron. 2003. "Symptom Improvement and Length of Treatment in Ethnically Similar and Dissimilar Client-Therapist Pairings." *Journal of Counseling Psychology* 50(1): 52–58.

Farmer, Paul. 2003. *Pathologies of Power.* Berkeley: University of California Press.

Flaskerud, Jacqueline H., and P. Y. Liu. 1991. "Effects of an Asian Client-Therapist Language, Ethnicity and Gender Match on Utilization and Outcome of Therapy." *Community Mental Health Journal* 27(1): 31–42.

Fujino, Diane C., Sumie Okazaki, and Kathleen Young. 1994. "Asian-American Women in the Mental Health System: An Examination of Ethnic and Gender Match Between Therapist and Client." *Journal of Community Psychology* 22(2): 164–76.

Good, Mary-Jo DelVecchio. 1995a. *American Medicine: The Quest for Competence.* Berkeley: University of California Press.

———. 1995b. "Cultural Studies of Biomedicine: An Agenda for Research." *Social Science & Medicine* 41(4): 461–73.

————. 2010. "The Medical Imaginary and the Biotechnical Embrace: Subjective Experiences of Clinical Scientists and Patients." In *A Reader in Medical Anthropology: Theoretical Trajectories, Emergent Realities,* edited by Byron J. Good, Michael M. J. Fischer, Sarah S. Willen, and Mary-Jo DelVecchio Good. Malden, Mass.: Wiley-Blackwell.

Good, Mary-Jo DelVecchio, and Byron J. Good. 2000. "Clinical Narratives and the Study of Contemporary Doctor-Patient Relationships." In *Handbook of Social Studies in Health and Medicine,* edited by Gary L. Albrecht, Ray Fitzpatrick, and Susan C. Scrimshaw. Thousand Oaks, Calif.: Sage Publications.

Good, Mary-Jo DelVecchio, Tseunetsugu Munakata, Yasuki Kobayashi, Cheryl Mattingly, Byron J. Good. 1994. "Oncology and Narrative Time." *Social Science & Medicine* 38(6): 855–62.

Hirsch, Jennifer S. 2003. "Anthropologists, Migrants, and Health Research: Confronting Cultural Appropriateness." In *American Arrivals: Anthropology Engages the New Immigration,* edited by Nancy Foner. Santa Fe, N.M.: SAR Press.

Jerrell, Jeanette M. 1995. "The Effects of Client-Therapist Match on Service Use and Costs." *Administration and Policy in Mental Health and Mental Health Services Research* 23(2): 119–26.

Jones, Enrico E. 1978. "Effects of Race on Psychotherapy Process and Outcome: An Exploratory Investigation." *Psychotherapy: Theory, Research, and Practice* 15(3): 226–36.

————. 1982. "Psychotherapists' Impressions of Treatment Outcome as a Function of Race." *Journal of Clinical Psychology* 38(4): 722–31.

Karlsson, Roger. 2005. "Ethnic Matching Between Therapist and Patient in Psychotherapy: An Overview of Findings, Together with Methodological and Conceptual Issues." *Cultural Diversity and Ethnic Minority Psychology* 11(2): 113–29.

Kirmayer, Laurence J. 2000. "Broken Narratives: Clinical Encounters and the Poetics of Illness Experience." In *Narrative and the Cultural Construction of Illness and Healing,* edited by Cheryl Mattingly and Linda Garro. Berkeley: University of California Press.

Kleinman, Arthur. 1988. *The Illness Narratives: Suffering, Healing, and the Human Condition.* New York: Basic Books.

————. 2006. *What Really Matters: Living a Moral Life Amidst Uncertainty and Danger.* New York: Oxford University Press.

Kleinman, Arthur, and Peter Benson. 2006. "Anthropology in the Clinic: The Problem of Cultural Competency and How to Fix It." *PLoS Medicine* 3(10): e294. Available at: http://www.plosmedicine.org/article/info%3Adoi%2F10. 1371%2Fjournal.pmed.0030294 (accessed June 24, 2011).

Kleinman, Arthur, Leon Eisenberg, and Byron J. Good. 1978. "Culture, Illness and Care." *Annals of Internal Medicine* 88(2): 251–58.

Lakes, Kimberly, Steven R. López, and Linda C. Garro. 2006. "Cultural Competence and Psychotherapy: Applying Anthropologically Informed Conceptions of Culture." *Psychotherapy: Theory, Research, Practice, and Training* 43(4): 380–96.

Liggan, Deborah Y., and Jerald Kay. 1999. "Race in the Room: Issues in the Dynamic Psychotherapy of African Americans." *Transcultural Psychiatry* 36(2): 195–209.

Maramba, Gloria Gia, and Gordon C. Nagayama Hall. 2002. "Meta-Analyses of Ethnic Match as a Predictor of Dropout, Utilization, and Level of Functioning." *Cultural Diversity and Ethnic Minority Psychology* 8(3): 290–97.

Mathews, Carol A., David Glidden, Stephen Murray, Peter Forster, and William A. Hargreaves. 2002. "The Effect on Treatment Outcomes of Assigning Patients to Ethnically Focused Inpatient Psychiatric Units." *Psychiatric Services* 53(7): 830–35.

Mattingly, Cheryl. 1994. "The Concept of Therapeutic 'Emplotment'." *Social Science and Medicine* 38(6): 811–22.

————. 1998. "In Search of the Good: Narrative Reasoning in Clinical Practice." *Medical Anthropology Quarterly* 12(3): 273–97.

Mattingly, Cheryl, and Linda C. Garro. 2000. *Narrative and the Cultural Construction of Illness and Healing*. Berkeley: University of California Press.

Ngai, Mae M. 2004. *Impossible Subjects: Illegal Aliens and the Making of Modern America*. Princeton, N.J.: Princeton University Press.

Proctor, Enola K., and Aaron Rosen. 1981. "Expectations and Preferences for Counselor Race and Their Relation to Intermediate Treatment Outcomes." *Journal of Counseling Psychology* 28(1): 40–46.

Ricker, Michael, Michael Nystul, and Michael Waldo. 1999. "Counselor and Clients' Ethnic Similarity and Therapeutic Alliance in Time-Limited Outcomes of Counseling." *Psychological Reports* 84(2): 674–76.

Rosenheck, Robert, and Catherine Leda Seibyl. 1998. "Participation and Outcome in a Residential Treatment and Work Therapy Program for Addictive Disorder: The Effects of Race." *American Journal of Psychiatry* 155(8): 1029–34.

Shin, Sung-Man, Clifton Chow, Teresita Camacho-Gonsalves, Rachel J. Levy, Elaine I. Allen, and Stephen H. Leff. 2005. "A Meta-Analytic Review of Racial-Ethnic Matching for African American and Caucasian American Clients and Clinicians." *Journal of Counseling Psychology* 52(1): 45–56.

Snowden, Lonnie R., Teh-wei Hu, and Jeanette M. Jerrell. 1995. Emergency Care Avoidance: Ethnic Matching and Participation in Minority-Serving Programs. *Community Mental Health Journal* 31(5): 463–73.

Sue, Stanley. 1998. "In Search of Cultural Competence in Psychotherapy and Counseling." *American Psychologist* 53(4):440–48.

————. 2003. "In Defense of Cultural Competency in Psychotherapy and Treatment." *American Psychologist* 58(11): 964–70.

Sue, Stanley, Diane C. Fujino, Li-tze Hu, David T. Takeuchi, Nolan W. S. Zane. 1991. "Community Mental Health Services for Ethnic Minority Groups: A Test of the Cultural Responsiveness Hypothesis." *Journal of Consulting and Clinical Psychology* 59(4): 533–40.

Sue, Stanley, and Nolan W. S. Zane. 1987. "The Role of Culture and Cultural Techniques in Psychotherapy: A Critique and Reformulation." *American Psychologist* 42(1): 37–45.

Takeuchi, David T., Stanley Sue, and May Yeh. 1995. "Return Rates and Outcomes from Ethnicity-Specific Mental Health Programs in Los Angeles." *American Journal of Public Health* 85(5): 638–43.

Terrell, Francis, and Sandra L. Terrell. 1984. "Race of Counselor, Client Sex, Cultural Mistrust Level, and Premature Termination from Counseling Among Black Clients." *Journal of Counseling Psychology* 31(3): 371–75.

Waters, Mary C. 1999. *Black Identities: West Indian Immigrant Dreams and American Realities.* New York: Russell Sage Foundation / Cambridge, Mass.: Harvard University Press.

Watkins, C. Edward, Jr., and Francis Terrell. 1988. "Mistrust Level and Its Effects on Counseling Expectations in Black Client-White Counselor Relationships: An Analogue Study." *Journal of Counseling Psychology* 35(2): 194–97.

Watkins, C. Edward, Jr., Francis Terrell, Fayneese S. Miller, and Sandra L. Terrell. 1989. "Cultural Mistrust and Its Effects on Expectational Variables in Black Client-White Counselor Relationships." *Journal of Counseling Psychology* 36(4): 447–50.

Zane, Nolan, Stanley Sue, Janet Chang, Lillian Huang, John Huang, Susana Lowe, Shobha Srinivasan, Kevin Chun, Karen Kurasaki, and Evelyn Lee. 2005. "Beyond Ethnic Match: Effects of Client-Therapist Cognitive Match in Problem Perception, Coping Orientation, and Therapy Goals on Treatment Outcomes." *Journal of Community Psychology* 33(5): 569–85.

Part II

Clinical Cultures,
Clinical Realities

T HE SIX chapters in "Clinical Cultures, Clinical Realities" reach into the heart of our project's investigations. The authors bring a unique mix of insider and outsider experiences and perspectives to their chapters. Antonio Bullon, Lawrence Park, and Marina Yaroshenko are psychiatrists in academic clinical practice, on the front lines providing care and directing clinics and services; they speak from inside the profession and as researchers of the profession. Joseph Calabrese and Sadeq Rahimi are anthropologists and also trained psychotherapists. Elizabeth Carpenter-Song, a psychological anthropologist, has extensive research experience with patients with psychiatric diagnoses. Sarah Willen, an anthropologist with a special interest in the health vulnerabilities associated with immigration, and Seth Hannah,[1] a sociologist specializing in inequality, race and ethnic relations, and cultural studies of medicine, whose field research brought us the concept of cultural environments of hyperdiversity, bring innovative theoretical perspectives from their disciplines and previous field work to the analyses of clinical cultures and clinical realities. Mary-Jo DelVecchio Good, principal investigator and designer of the project, is a comparative sociologist and medical anthropologist with three decades of teaching, research, and writing on culture, medicine, and psychiatry, and on the culture of medicine in the United States and internationally.

Culture counts in these chapters. When we asked clinicians and healthcare staff, "Does culture matter in mental health care? And in what ways, in your practice, in your institution?" discussions easily unfolded, with much talk about culture. Culture was everywhere, and sometimes nowhere. Those interviewed explained ways they and their clinic, hospital, or service respond to the complex cultural diversity of patient populations they serve. They also spoke about the cultures of their own clinics and of treatment models, and about the culture of co-workers in terms of race, ethnicity, language, national origin, immigration status, religion, and gender. Some discussed major cultural distinctions within psychiatry, contrasting biological and neurological models of illness and treatment with those dominated by pharmacological and medication models, and with psychodynamic talk therapy, often now a rarity. Clinicians also spoke about how they go beyond bounded notions of culture to ideas of universalism, to establish trust with individual patients, "breast to breast, chest to chest," about humanism and seeing the patient as a person. Patients interviewed also spoke about cultures of clinical practice, assessing the positive and negative aspects encountered. If one thinks of 'culture' as a star burst—shattered into many parts and meanings but still there—it resembles the culture talk in the interviews that provide the empirical grounding for these chapters.

An unsettling theme runs through these chapters as well. Psychiatrists, from senior attendings and leaders in the field to young residents and trainees, readily spoke of their concerns about the future of psychiatry and their ability to fulfill their soteriological[2] mission to provide care to the mentally ill, regardless of their culture. One leading clinician said that he was worried about "the disappearance of thoughtfulness regarding issues of culture and the importance of making a relationship with patients." Others expressed frustration and irritation at the intrusion on therapeutic activities of newly burgeoning documentation practices required for quality assurance, insurance coverage, patient rights, and patient records. Many clinicians experience these changes as impediments to providing appropriate and culturally tailored, sensitive care to the poor, to new immigrants, and to non-English-speaking patients in need. These comments also reflect clinicians' experience of an assault on their professional power and cultural authority, their disappearing control over the nature of their work.

Chapter 6, "Portrait of a Psychiatrist," by Sarah Willen, Marina Yaroshenko, Seth Hannah, Ken Vickery, and Mary-Jo DelVecchio Good, is a collaborative effort that emerged from a series of interviews with a Soviet-educated physician we call Dr. Z. The chapter traces two parallel journeys. First, it follows Dr. Z.'s personal journey from Kazakhstan, where her parents—both psychiatrists—held medical posts, to Latvia, where she trained as a physician, and through a difficult process of emigration and professional recertification in the United States. This personal trajectory is entwined with Dr. Z.'s professional journey through multiple schools of psychiatry in the Soviet Union and in the United States, where she pursued residency training just as psychoanalytic approaches were rapidly disappearing from academic hospital residency training programs and being usurped by biological models of diagnosis and treatment.

Dr. Z.'s complex narrative shatters any simple or bounded definition of culture either for psychiatry, for clinics, for patients, or for herself. Torn between a sense that psychiatry holds universal promise, on one hand, and a competing sense that linguistic obstacles and cultural difference can interfere with the profession's capacity to serve patients, she is ambivalent about the impact of techniques discussed in part I, such as clinician-patient matching, medical interpretation, and cultural competence training.

The sense of unease Dr. Z. articulates concerning the identity or culture of contemporary psychiatry resonates with chapter 7, "Psychiatry in a Flat World," by Sadeq Rahimi, Seth Hannah, and Mary-Jo DelVecchio Good. The authors illustrate how psychiatry is not a closed culture, but shaped instead by many external factors, including a growing cosmopolitanism associated with the increasing hyperdiversity of patient populations. The senior clinicians interviewed for this chapter speak about how they approach patients, not with a reductive stance of "I know you" (that is, your culture, background, race, ethnicity), but instead with a more individualistic approach, asking, "Who are you?" Patient culture, to these clinicians, does not necessarily mean racial and ethnic identity; it also means recognizing other forms of cultural distinction considered important to building a therapeutic alliance. The inpatient service at this research site is notable for not being exclusive, for being able "to treat anybody from any culture." With new treatment modalities based on medication therapies, patients no longer need be proficient in English to be admitted.

These findings resonate with Elizabeth Carpenter-Song's analysis in chapter 8, "Recognition in Clinical Relationships." Reporting with some astonishment that in contrast to her previous research with psychiatric patients, many of whom felt that "doctors don't treat you like a person," she finds that patients she interviewed for this study had positive experiences with their treatment. Patients represented a mélange of race, ethnicity, gender, class and age, illustrative of American institutions of cultural hyperdiversity. Carpenter-Song asks, "What is one to make of happy patients?" Identifying the importance of patient voices and the quality of clinician voices, and drawing on Judith Butler's notion of recognition, Carpenter-Song urges that the question "who are you?" is critical to making therapeutic alliances in mental health care, regardless of patient culture. She concludes noting the positive dynamics of recognition in therapeutic work are contingent on a political economy of care that allows for patients and clinicians to be "good." Her warnings of the fragile balance between following insurers' rules and providing what the patient needs in the context of an academic inpatient unit echo the struggles of psychiatrists serving non-English-speaking minorities in less well-funded outpatient settings.

In chapter 9, "'The Culture of Medicine' As Revealed in Patients' Perspectives on Psychiatric Treatment," Joseph Calabrese explores the culture of medicine through an analysis of ways psychiatric patients describe negative and positive clinical encounters. He argues that the depersonalized medical gaze and bureaucratic practices of contemporary medicine pose barriers to quality therapeutic relationships. Like Carpenter-Song and the senior psychiatrists discussed earlier, he identifies that recognizing the patient as a person makes—from the patient perspective—for good therapeutic relationships. Depersonalization and "being treated like a specimen" leads to distrust not only in an individual clinician but also perhaps of an entire institution and professional discipline. The interviews Calabrese discusses illustrate the same multiple dimensions of culture Hannah notes in his concept of hyperdiversity. Cultural difference can be a relevant barrier for white patients as well, particularly those within minority religious traditions. In addition, interviews with patients reveal that carrying the stigma of mental illness also has cultural dimensions. Calabrese argues that both patients and therapists see burgeoning bureaucratic practices (documentation) as encroaching on clinicians' listening, communicating, and recognizing time. And institutional efforts to ethnically match patients and clinicians (see chapter 5, this volume)—itself a new aspect of the culture of medicine—will miss these subtler forms of cultural difference and complicate efforts to build positive therapeutic relationships.

Calabrese's argument and findings resonate with chapter 10, "The Paper Life of Minority and Low-Income Patient Care," by Antonio Bullon, Good, and Carpenter-Song. This chapter uses two unique sets of interviews; first, interviews by Bullon with clinicians who work in academic medical center outpatient clinics, including a Latino clinic that serves both Spanish-speaking and poor or low-income patients; and second, narrative reflections by the psychiatrist Bullon, initially expressed orally in a series of interviews with Mary-Jo DelVecchio Good. Following Donald Schon's (1983) method of the reflective practitioner, we enter the field through the psychiatrist's account of a Monday morning at the Latino clinic. Through vivid scenarios (again originally conveyed in Good's interviews with Bullon), we are presented with unfolding layers of the paper life—a life that expands and intrudes on clinic time and therapeutic work with patients. These scenarios have an undercurrent of humor in the recounting, in part because of the absurdity of some of the templates and documentation practices. Yet the authors ask what the implication is of the expansion of a paper life "that does not fit the complexities of clinical practice or patient life," that deletes clinically meaningful data, eliding the social complexities of patients and the therapeutic actions and assessments of the clinicians. The chapter argues that the culture of clinical work has been transformed through an expansion of documentation practices meeting the needs of managed care and quality assurance and concludes with recommendations for making documentation practices clinically relevant and useful.

Chapter 11, "Physicians' Perspectives on Financial Barriers to Equitable Care," by Seth Hannah, Lawrence Park, and Mary-Jo DelVecchio Good, highlights the experiences of mental health clinicians and clinic directors with a maze of insurance and financial regulations. Clinicians have vivid ways of describing managing and going through the maze. Visceral reactions are evoked when clinicians speak about "patients churning, clinics dumping," and everyone getting "stuck" in the financial maze. They lament the loss of free care, and though they appreciate the intent to provide universal coverage, they experience the maze as undercutting their professional and cultural authority. As we analyzed the interviews using Atlas.ti, finding many discussions of finance and insurance, we asked ourselves whether economy would trump culture. Our findings suggest that cultural projects, policies, and programs are readily taken up by most clinicians, excluding occasional residents who do not want their cultural knowledge "technologized." However, these activities should not be seen in a vacuum; we also found that the financial considerations and the political economy of care significantly complicate efforts to provide equitable care to racial, ethnic, and cultural minorities.

This chapter foregrounds one of the central insights of this book: although cultural diversity poses substantial challenges to psychiatry and medicine, it does so in nuanced and complicated ways that include multiple dimensions of difference (hyperdiversity). These multiple dimensions of cultural difference, including social class and immigration and refugee status, interact with larger structural forces in the way health care is organized and financed—determining whether a patient can be admitted to inpatient treatment or is eligible for publicly funded health insurance to pay for needed medications. Thus the political economy of care may not completely trump culture, but it does shatter any assumption that patient culture can be adequately addressed without considering the broader cultures of psychiatry, American medicine, and American society.

Notes

1. For Hannah, the concept of *cultural environments of hyperdiversity* emerged directly out of his ethnographic field research in several clinics and services, first as my project research assistant and then as a Ph.D. candidate in the Department of Sociology at Harvard University, undertaking dissertation research as part of this larger project.

2. According to *Webster's Dictionary* (1912), *soteriological* is defined as: "1) A discourse on health or hygiene and 2) *Theol.* The doctrine of salvation by Jesus Christ" (1997). (See also Good 1994.) *Soteriological* is used here to denote the affective and moral dimensions of doctoring, the sense of higher meaning derived from taking care of others.

References

Good, Byron J. 1994. *Medicine, Rationality, and Experience: An Anthropological Perspective.* Cambridge: Cambridge University Press.

Schon, Donald. 1983. *The Reflective Practitioner.* New York: Basic Books.

Webster's New International Dictionary of the English Language. 1912. Springfield, Mass.: G&C Merriam Company.

Chapter 6

Portrait of a Psychiatrist

SARAH S. WILLEN, MARINA YAROSHENKO,
SETH DONAL HANNAH, KEN VICKERY,
AND MARY-JO DELVECCHIO GOOD

Like if you ask me, I personally think I do a lot of things against my culture, and I would not consider myself your typical Latvian, or Russian; immigrant, or psychiatrist. Now ... of course I have a lot of characteristics— I have the same accent that they can't get rid of, or mannerisms, or certain things, but back over there, I consider myself as an out—what's the word?—outsider? Or out—the one that does not fit in to the culture. So if you try to think, all right, "I understand the Russian culture," and not, "I am going to treat her"—let's say I'm your patient—"based on her culture," you'll make a mistake.

—Dr. Z.

AS THESE personal reflections from Dr. Z. suggest, the tendency within American biomedicine to advance a model of culturally competent care conceals a not-so-hidden possibility of misguided—and misleading—presumption, assumption, and stereotyping. Our overall study findings suggest these forms of stereotyping— especially when they intersect with increasing pressures toward efficiency, routinization, bureaucratization, and legalistic defensiveness— often interfere with clinicians' professional mandate to approach each patient as a unique person who desires, and indeed deserves, personalized clinical attention.

In this chapter, we explore these distancing tendencies from the perspective of Dr. Z., a Soviet-trained psychiatrist who, after completing her clinical training, immigrated to the United States under difficult circumstances; pursued a lengthy and challenging process of professional retraining and recertification; and reoriented herself to the rapidly changing medical culture of her new country. We draw heavily upon two extended interviews in which this psychiatrist—who is both a practicing clinician and an integral part of our research team—spoke at length about her understanding of how culture counts in contemporary American psychiatric practice. As someone who immigrated to the United States herself and struggled to learn a new language, acclimate to a new culture, and reground her sense of personal and professional identity, Dr. Z. brings a unique perspective to the constellation of contemporary challenges at the center of our study.

This chapter is organized around four key themes. First, we consider how this particular psychiatrist's personal biography—including her experiences of choosing a career in psychiatry and of immigrating to the United States—have shaped her sense of professional identity. We then explore the multiple, divergent models of psychiatric practice she has encountered over the course of her clinical career. With her unique but illustrative biography as backdrop, we then consider some of her struggles to negotiate differences of culture and language in her clinical work. In concluding, we return to a core dilemma for Dr. Z: How can mental health care providers acknowledge shared dimensions of cultural identity and yet approach each patient as a unique human being, remembering that beyond diverse and competing therapeutic models there is, as Dr. Z. observes, a person behind the patient?

Choosing Psychiatry

For Dr. Z., choosing a career in psychiatry enabled her not only to become part of a professional world that attracted her interest and curiosity but also, in effect, to join the family business. Born in the former Soviet Union to highly educated, highly mobile parents—both of whom were themselves psychiatrists—she was initially attracted to other professional paths, but eventually made the choice to follow in their footsteps. "I was always fascinated by . . . languages. And maybe some romantic streak in me, I wanted to travel, I wanted to see the world. I was curious about other cultures, how other people live. My mother at that time . . . said, 'You know, you can study languages on your own, but you need to have job,' which is how I ended up here."

Her choice to study first medicine and then psychiatry were deeply influenced by the intellectual climate that surrounded her as a child and young adult. Many of her parents' friends were psychiatrists, and together they spoke

> about interesting patients, maybe talking about some ideas, some thoughts, so I was exposed to all that, indirectly. The first time I was trying to make

a decision . . . I thought maybe gynecology. But then you have to be a surgeon, and it's very, the lifestyle I didn't like. Or maybe internal medicine. But again, it wasn't that interesting, and on top of it, I thought, well, maybe I should use the opportunity that my parents know everybody within the system so it will actually be easier for me to get through the system.

Although her innate curiosity, combined with her parents' professional connections, proved helpful in the earliest stages of her career, she first had to obtain high scores on a national matriculation exam and then on a biology exam. Dr. Z. felt these examinations—difficult in their own right—were especially challenging because she had received substandard education in Kazakhstan, where her father was posted as a military physician when Dr. Z. was in elementary school. It was after her family moved from Kazakhstan to Riga, Latvia, during her teenage years that she was able to catch up to the level of better-prepared students from more developed areas of the Soviet Union.

During the first stage of Dr. Z.'s clinical training in Latvia in the mid-1980s, Soviet psychiatry was deeply influenced by German organic psychiatric theories; institutionalization for the mentally ill was a long-term prospect; and talk therapy—Freudian or otherwise—was virtually anathema. She graduated from medical school after completing the standard six years of medical training and after submitting a final paper that captured the spirit of Soviet psychiatry at the time: "Why Freudian Theory Is Wrong."

Immigration to the United States: Opportunities and Obstacles

Within a few years after completing her medical training, Dr. Z. and her parents—influenced by family friends—made a decision that was not only difficult, but also risky in both professional and personal terms. They decided to apply for permission to leave the Soviet Union. Although emigration was generally prohibited by the Soviet authorities, one exit pathway opened up in the mid-1980s for a limited group of Soviet citizens: individuals of Jewish descent and their families. Because Dr. Z.'s mother was Jewish, the three of them would be eligible to emigrate if they could obtain an invitation to Israel from a relative. Although they were able to arrange such an invitation, the opportunity to ask permission to leave came at a steep price:

> You would go through hell basically, and a lot of people did . . . because if you happened to be in a decent position at work, you would be fired, and also you would be exposed to the meeting when everybody would present what a bad person you are. Now you want to leave the country that gave you so much, and on and on. So there's a lot of shame. . . . You're also taking a risk because you may end up not being allowed to

leave, and then you have to live with the consequences, so to speak. So we did the same thing, basically, when Gorbachev came to power.

When Dr. Z. and her parents filed an application to leave in 1987, she was twenty-six and her parents were in their early fifties. Upon leaving the Soviet Union, they had to turn in their passports and leave only with "$120 and two suitcases, basically. Some people were able to send the furniture, but we didn't. We were like, two suitcases per person and that's it, basically. So it was a pretty traumatic process."

Her family's immigration process was further complicated when her mother was diagnosed with breast cancer in the year before their departure. "My mother went to the hospital, and my father and I basically started to get ready. We did have this dilemma of maybe staying and her getting treatment or maybe basics and then leaving, so that she would get treatment here [in the United States]. And she did have a surgery and a radiation there and then we left."

Although Dr. Z. and her family had initially thought about moving to Australia, her mother's diagnosis led them to change their plans and instead make the safer choice of emigrating to the United States, where they knew they would have a stronger network of support. "Because of my mother's illness and no guarantees," she explained, "I knew she needed some treatment, so we just couldn't take chances. Basically from that point, her illness colored the whole immigration experience."

In the United States, however, neither Dr. Z. nor her parents were able to work as physicians. Her mother was too ill to work, and both Dr. Z. and her father lacked the appropriate recertification. Initially she found work as an interpreter and an assistant social worker. Her father worked as a taxi driver until he found work at a medical device company and later retrained as a registered nurse. Eventually they decided as a family that too many obstacles, among them age and limited English skills, would prevent her father from repeating his medical training in the United States, but that Dr. Z. would. Just as she began to prepare for the United States Medical Licensing Examination (USMLE), her mother succumbed to breast cancer. In the years that followed, Dr. Z. plunged into her studies, re-learned in English all she had originally learned in Russian, passed the USMLE exam with a high score—and began to search for a residency training program.

The Cultures of Psychiatry

When Dr. Z. interviewed for residency programs in the early 1990s, American psychiatry was at a critical turning point. After psychoanalysis' long reign, newer, biologically based models of brain function were gaining rapid ascendance, and psychodynamic models of diagnosis and "talk therapy" had been deeply shaken if not yet fully usurped by a new biological focus on brain function and pharmaceutical treatment (Luhrmann 2000). Although she initially joined a biologically inclined residency program, Dr. Z. quickly determined it a poor fit and transferred to a program in which she initially had taken little interest: a renowned psychiatric hospital with an unwavering commitment to psychodynamic models of mental health treatment.

It was in this unique, once-radical clinical environment, more than at any other stage of her clinical training, that Dr. Z. felt psychiatry was at its best. Although the program, too, had begun to capitulate to the prevailing pressures of the late-twentieth-century American health-care system, she nonetheless felt that

> choosing [that] program was one of the best moves I made in my entire life. . . . It was open, it was very supportive, very nurturing, a different way to approach people, treat people. It was much more—[in] hindsight it was the way intuitively I felt would be the right way. When I just started, people were not wearing badges. You mix with the patients, basically. Go to [the] cafeteria, you don't know who is the patient, who is the staff. Which I thought was fascinating, it was great. But towards when I was leaving, they implemented the badge system, and by then the staff was wearing badges. And unfortunately, I went through this whole process of watching [the hospital] going down the hill, in a way. . . . At that time, I was still focused on [how] we're all human, and we're not that different from the patient. It was a really nice philosophy.

Dr. Z.'s enthusiasm stemmed in part from the hospital's psychoanalytic inclinations, which were worlds apart from both the Soviet psychiatry in which she was trained and the biological model that was already taking hold in the U.S. residency program she initially joined and quickly left.

More than the theory itself, however, she saw value in how theoretical commitments to psychoanalysis were translated into the messy and complicated world of holistic therapeutic practice:

> Whatever they were teaching just fell into the right spot in me. Mostly it was psychodynamic principles, but those people were really practicing it. They really cared about the patients, they really saw patients as human. That's probably, the way patients [were] treated was the best, in the sense [that] there was no separation. And also promoting the growth, really talking about [patients'] growth. And really having time and place to stop and think and process and care for each other. So there was this environment of staff caring for each other, and then we all cared for the patients. And I liked that. . . . I haven't seen that anywhere else. I tried to give it to residents when I was supervising here.

As she advanced from trainee to attending physician and moved to Boston, Dr. Z. took these core values with her and integrated them into her subsequent teaching, clinical practice, and evolving sense of professional identity.

As a practicing clinician and a clinical instructor, Dr. Z. has worked in a wide variety of clinical environments, each of them worlds away from the warm, supportive atmosphere—both for patients, she noted, and for clinical staff—in which she completed her residency. Her more recent places of employment have included a large academic hospital, several small community health centers, and a psychiatric facility for individuals court-ordered to receive mental health assessment and care. None of these treatment settings follows the holistic psychodynamic model that Dr. Z. found so deeply appealing; all privilege psychopharmacology over psychotherapy, place constraints on the time clinicians can spend with patients, and subject clinicians to the combined demands of DSM-IV-based diagnostic precision and administrative bureaucracy. What all of these clinical settings share—some of them inpatient, some outpatient; some large, some small; some supportive and encouraging for patients and others paternalistic and forensically minded—is the increasing diversity within their patient populations associated with broader changes taking place in the Boston metropolitan era including, in particular, growing hyperdiversity.

Culture in the Clinic: Does It Matter?

Like many of the clinicians we interviewed, Dr. Z. described herself as feeling torn between a sense that psychiatry holds universal promise for all who have mental health concerns, even as cultural difference and linguistic obstacles can limit the profession's ability to serve its patients. What she can articulate with confidence, however, is a sense that reductionist models of cultural competence are more harmful to clinicians and clinicians-in-training than they are helpful. As an alternative—and influenced, to a large extent, by her residency experience—she advocates a holistic clinical approach in which the clinician strives to make sense of a patient's psychiatric distress within the broader context of his or her unique lifeworld. In key respects, Dr. Z.'s clinical orientation resonates with the recommendations of medical anthropologists and clinicians who exhort health care providers to initiate clinical relationships by first conducting mini-ethnographies that might help them maximize their understanding of their patients' unique lifeworlds (Kleinman 1988; Kleinman and Benson 2006; compare Lakes, López, and Garro 2006).

Cultural Background Versus Broader Life Context

This nuanced perspective emerged when we asked Dr. Z. about her views on cultural competence training. Her initial response was blunt, but then she clarified and softened her stance:

I think it's useless. No, that's not what I'm trying to say. I think you have to be really careful about it, and really thoughtful about applying stereotypes, and so many people have already said that. I believe in context. Call it the culture, call it the personal factors, call it objective experience. But I do believe that you have to take into consideration the context. And with some patients the context could be exactly [a] cultural stereotype. They would fit perfectly. And you would take . . . his next door neighbor in the same town, the same age, the same situation. And it would be a very different person. However, how do you know which one is which? You don't. . . . I still believe in that psychodynamic cliché question of, "What does it mean to you?" I think it's a very powerful question.

Dr. Z. has no doubt that cultural background and other external dimensions of a patient's life—for example, family context, immigrant status, socioeconomic class—shape his or her experiences of psychiatric distress. On the other hand, culture and cultural difference may be distant from the core issues she must understand if she hopes to craft an effective treatment plan for any specific patient. She articulates this point clearly in this chapter's opening quote, where she speaks hypothetically about how a psychiatrist might encounter her as a patient. A clinician might be tempted to reduce her, for example, to a stock notion of a typical Latvian, or Russian, or immigrant—or psychiatrist. In her view—itself sharpened on the whetstone of her own complicated personal biography—individuals do not blindly recapitulate the values or commitments of the environments in which they are raised.

These comments suggest two key insights. First, Dr. Z.'s recognition that individuals may simultaneously embody some elements of a culture but adamantly reject others implies a powerful critique of the kind of bluntly wielded, checklist-type models that often drive cultural competency training initiatives. Second, and more subtly, her self-reflective opening comment reveals the enduring influence of her distinctive residency training experience. Unlike many of the clinicians we interviewed, she comfortably turns the discursive table around and speaks from the hypothetical position of a patient. This subtle rhetorical move resonates with Dr. Z.'s observations earlier in the interviews about her deeply rooted commitment to the notion that clinicians and patients—although cast in opposing roles in the often adversarial drama of contemporary U.S. psychiatry—ultimately have more in common than is generally acknowledged. Behind the social masks of white coats and professionalized identities, diagnostic labels and sick roles, she contends, is nothing less than the common experience of being human.

Language Barriers

Although she is committed to the notion that clinicians and patients share more than what divides them, Dr. Z. spoke frankly about the formidable obstacles that can erode a clinician's capacities for compassion and empathy—including her own. In Dr. Z.'s experience, more often it is not cultural difference but rather barriers of language that can wall patients off from the benefits of a clinician's personalized professional concern. As a clinician who sees patients both in English, which she speaks with eloquent fluency, and in her native Russian, the patients who challenge Dr. Z. most are (non-Russian speaking) immigrants to the United States with limited English proficiency (LEP).

Dr. Z. acknowledged that medical interpreters, who play an increasingly prominent role in U.S. health-care settings, are important resources for her and her colleagues (see chapter 3, this volume). According to the interpreters we interviewed, the success or failure of interpreted encounters hinges, to a large extent, on a clinician's appreciation of the interpreter's role and his or her level of comfort working with a linguistic mediator. One issue our interpreter-interviewees failed to note, however, was among the first that Dr. Z. mentioned when the issue of LEP patients arose: time pressure. She explained in strikingly honest terms what runs through her mind when she becomes responsible for a patient with whom she may not share a common language:

> I see the foreign name, and I'm already dreading it, because if that's going to be an immigrant, a foreign patient, I know it's going to be a mess. The reality is, it's probably going to take me [an] extra two hours and I'm going to be late for my next job, and it's going to make my work life more difficult. This is the basic practical reality of it. Because I have to call [an] interpreter, I have to schedule the time, I have to have all these people involved, I have to talk to the family to understand what's going on. . . . It takes so much more time.

In such instances, Dr. Z.'s mind races ahead to the communicative, diagnostic, technical, and bureaucratic challenges she is likely to confront. Once she notices that an upcoming patient has a "foreign name," she explains, "I see the name, then my next step, I would ask the, whoever is around, do they speak English?" If the clinical team member answers in the affirmative, "it's like 'Phew!' . . . Like [that's] at least three-quarters of the problem." If the patient does not speak English, however, "I think, oh gosh, no, my day is not going to go as I was hoping it was going to go." Under circumstances like these—and despite her desire to seek out "the person behind the patient" and her acute awareness of the challenges immigrants face in unfamiliar health care systems—Dr. Z. is automatically driven to think practically. Practically speaking, and despite hospitals' efforts to make interpretation services more readily available, the clinical environments in which she works cannot easily accommodate the lengthier consultation times that become necessary when language constitutes a barrier to clinical care.

Sometimes a consultation is delayed because no medical interpreter is immediately available. Sometimes interpretation is available, but only through a telephone interpretation service. Dr. Z. explained that even the few minutes required to set up a phone interpretation can be disruptive when she is responsible for a long list of patients on a busy unit:

> I had this Chinese lady, a couple of months ago, on [an inpatient ward at an academic hospital]. She was very quiet; she didn't talk much; she had ECT [electroconvulsive therapy]; the husband was involved. She did not speak any English. . . . We had to use the interpreter machine [a telephone built for conference calls]. But even that, that one or two extra minutes to wheel that thing in . . . It's still a few more minutes. Because you have to call, you have to get that interpreter, you have to start talking, it's cumbersome, it's complicated . . . All this wait and you only have two hours to do the rounds and you need to get it done and there are all the other things to do.

In this case, all Dr. Z. needed to ask of the patient were a few straightforward questions: "'How is your appetite? How is your sleep? How is your energy? How [are] any side effects?' That's it."[1] Although this vignette may revolve around a series of minor disruptions, it nonetheless provides a telling illustration of how clinicians, and the American healthcare system writ large, are struggling to confront the diverse implications of the country's growing hyperdiversity.

Cultural Knowledge: When, and How, Does It Matter?

Despite Dr. Z.'s overarching commitment to the notion that shared humanity outweighs shared culture in facilitating effective clinical communication, she acknowledged that nuanced cultural and linguistic knowledge can, at times, be critical to the process of diagnosis and treatment. For instance, she described a recent consultation with a Russian patient in his eighties in which her task was to determine whether he was psychotic or delirious:

> So I come to see this man. Among other things, he says, "You know, weird thing, like I'm usually normal and then suddenly I would have, like there is a wall and there is clock and suddenly everything is on the floor and I am in a vertical position and I feel like my bed is vertical. And it lasts [a] certain amount of time, and then it goes away."

As her consultation with the older man unfolded, Dr. Z. understood why a clinician relying on a partial understanding of his words—and, more fundamentally, of his illness phenomenology—might have suspected psychosis or delirium. However, she grew increasingly convinced that the clinical portrait he described mapped the neurological effects of Parkinson's disease:

> And then he also tells me, "You know what? I keep track of all the dates, I try to remember this" and so he, and I wonder how much in this interaction, the culture mattered. Because I could see clearly he was not psychotic. And that hallucinations seemed to be clearly the neurological [impact] due to Parkinson's, some kind of seizures, because he can explain that so clearly and he was very aware of what's going on . . . but I think this is not a cultural issue. That was the language issue.

In this particular instance, Dr. Z.'s fluency in Russian made it possible to quickly develop a differential diagnosis that excluded psychiatric conditions and suggested a neurological condition instead. Here, it was language that mattered; had her patient seen a non-Russian-speaking clinician, an effective interpreter could have helped bridge the gap.

On some occasions, however, culture—even more than language—can impede the work of clinical care. For example, Dr. Z. recounted a case involving

> the family of an older man, ninety or something, not that demented, but he was again sick and delirious. And the daughter-in-law was very demanding. And as I started talking to social workers, they would roll their eyes and [talk about] how difficult she is. But to me, it's very clear why she's so difficult, because she is used to . . . [the] Soviet system, where you know that you have to take it into your own hands; you cannot trust the system.

For the social workers, this daughter-in-law's behavior signified excessive involvement, even meddling, in the work of the clinical team—and she annoyed them. Although Dr. Z. could understand the social workers' response, she also understood through personal experience that there was nothing peculiar about the daughter-in-law's behavior. Given the woman's experiences with the Soviet medical system, in which patients might get lost unless a relative took on the role of active and vocal advocate, she was simply acting as she thought a patient's caring relative should. Although Dr. Z. understood the daughter-in-law's motives, actions, and demands, for the rest of the staff she was "just really annoying," "too controlling," and "too demanding."

In this particular instance, Dr. Z. recognized that the cultural and political experience she shared with the patient and his family—an unplanned "cultural match"—served as a useful clinical resource. Yet she saw a flip side to this deep cultural familiarity as well:

> Because the other side of it, I . . . easily got sucked into it, so to speak. Into those dynamics, like, yes, let's say, I think I consulted maybe on three

Russian patients and two of them I spoke with, the daughter-in-law, the wife. And the wife started telling me how difficult it is for them . . . so I'm so drawn to start to be case manager for them, and then I get entangled in my own countertransference, so to speak. So on one hand, I understand them well, but do I help them? I don't know.

In fact, Dr. Z. wondered whether the cultural knowledge and experiences she shared with these patients might ultimately impede her efforts to provide good care. "I think sometimes I can really be of a lot of help. And sometimes I can maybe not be as helpful as somebody who does not know what they're coming from, and just treats them as, 'All right, I see this, this and that happening and that's how we treat it and that's what we're gonna do.'"

In other words, attention to specific dimensions of a patient's cultural background—at least in theory—can help clarify a diagnostic process, defuse tension between patients (or their relatives) and clinical staff, or develop a viable treatment plan. Under other circumstances, however, Dr. Z.'s reflections suggest that shared cultural knowledge—especially between immigrant patients and immigrant physicians of the same cultural background—might actually run the risk of impeding processes of treatment and care. Her insights thus deepen the argument we advanced earlier concerning the potential limitations of "matching" as a strategy for improving clinician-patient rapport (see chapter 5, this volume).

Clinical Strategies

During our conversations with Dr. Z., she continually turned our questions about culture, cultural difference, and clinical interactions over and over in her mind. We found it valuable to hear her wonder aloud about the relationship among questions of culture and clinical practice, her personal experience as an immigrant, and her familiarity and facility with so many different psychiatric cultures of theory and practice (among them Soviet psychiatry, American biological psychiatry, American psychoanalytic psychiatry, forensic psychiatry, and community-based mental health care). As we thought aloud together, it became increasingly clear that Dr. Z.—like her colleagues throughout the profession—is struggling to reconcile competing clinical demands within a rapidly changing professional context. How can she juggle the need to diagnose and treat, the need to appreciate patients in the holistic fullness of their lifeworlds or biopsychosocial contexts, the exhortations of the cultural competence models to which she and her profession have been exposed, and the profound practical challenges associated with growing diversity among her patients? As she reflected on these questions, Dr. Z. homed in on two favored clinical strategies that illustrate how her personal experience has influenced her professional responses to these challenges. One of these strategies is well suited to one-on-one clinical encounters, and the other is geared primarily toward the responsibilities of the attending physician in team-based clinical care environments.

Understanding What's in a Patient's "Bundle"

First, Dr. Z. finds great significance in a fellow clinician's observation that for some refugees, "the bundle of stuff that they brought from their country . . . just the junk that [someone else] would want to throw . . . in the garbage" is "everything. Their life. . . . I try to keep that in mind." As a clinician, Dr. Z. tries to "put my antenna out to be aware of" whatever it is that constitutes a patient's metaphoric "bundle" of prized possessions—or memories, or experiences, or relationships—and to begin engaging him or her through the lens of that "bundle." "And I'll be honest," she said,

> [it's] not that I'm always able to get it. But at least try to be open to the possibility that there is that bundle, you know. Whatever you call it, . . . like when you—[have an] apron, [in which] you put your most precious possessions, five most precious possessions. . . . If they do have them, I try to find out what they are. . . . To be open and try not to miss, if there is, call it a big elephant in the room, whatever, but whatever is important to them, and not to judge that . . . by the standard of society, or whatever common scale, so to speak. And try to get to them at that level, the issue specifically.

Sometimes Dr. Z. needs to learn more about a patient's culture to fully appreciate what's in the "bundle"; on other occasions, sincere interest and a sense of common humanity are enough to help her begin to see, understand, and connect with what she describes as "the person behind the patient."

Setting the Tone for a Clinical Care Team

What happens when a psychiatrist serves in a supervisory role for a large clinical team? Under the tight time constraints, insurance-related demands, and other institutional pressures of a busy urban hospital, how can an attending psychiatrist promote a model of care-giving that is nonetheless attentive to the person behind the patient? Under such circumstances, psychiatrists are far too busy to spend the kind of quiet hours with patients that Dr. Z. could spend in another kind of mental health care setting, in another time, and in another place. When she serves in this role, the strategy Dr. Z. strives to employ is quite simple; she strives to set a humanistic tone.

Curious but a bit perplexed, one of us [KV] pressed her for clarification. "Wait," he asked. "Is it psychiatrists that set this tone . . . or is it hospital administration? Or is it managed care in some big brother kind of way?

Or is it 'the system' in the broader sense of the word? I mean, who is it that actually sets this tone that you're talking about?" After a thoughtful moment, Dr. Z. elaborated, "I think it comes from above. So the system sets the tone, but then the psychiatrist can modulate."

She described several different clinical settings in which she had worked: first, a forensic mental health care center where "the system sets [a] very impersonal tone" and she "was trying to fight it and lost, basically;" second, a community hospital with a warm, team-like dynamic; and third, a large academic hospital where the words and actions of an attending psychiatrist can readily "set the tone" for a clinical team, a shift, or an entire unit. There, Dr. Z. explained, "when [the] psychiatrist is not interested, then the whole team's suffering." When she works at the academic hospital as attending psychiatrist, the clinical team

> is especially big. I have a resident, at least [one] resident, a social worker, the case manager, the nurse.... Plus, there [are] oftentimes student nurses, [a] student psychologist, sometimes the psychologist is present.... If I keep talking from the very impersonal view, they would not be feeling free to show that they can be personal.... If I noticed that this [is] all starting to be too impersonal, concerned too much about labs and drugs and levels and other systems, then I can throw [out] just one sentence: "Wait a second, did anybody talk to his wife?" for example. "Did anybody ask what's going on at home that he is that depressed?" Or like, "What's up with this situation? Can social work, can you please call, and can we look into that?" So just one question, and that already sets the whole team in a different direction.

In fact, Dr. Z. felt strongly that this sort of intervention is precisely what an attending psychiatrist is required to do: to invite other members of a mental health team to do what they are trained to do and, moreover, what they generally want to do. One of us [KV] pushed her for further clarification, suggesting that if mental health clinicians have been trained "within a rigid, impersonal system, it would be pretty difficult to steer them in the direction of a more personal, humanitarian type of care. But what you're saying is that a simple sentence can do it. So it tells me that they're primed to go in that direction anyway. Sort of waiting for the OK. Is that the case?"

Dr. Z. responded in the affirmative, suggesting that nurses and social workers—more than doctors—are expected to look for the person behind the patient. In her view, it is thus psychiatrists themselves—in part because of the ascendance of biological models and rigid diagnostic algorithms within psychiatry—who sometimes stand in the way of humane care. "Like the nurses, I think they have that [more humanitarian approach to care]. Just as the social workers. It's the doctors that, the problem is with us. We walk in trained to be the most impersonal. And that's why they just have to get your OK."

Conclusion

As this portrait reveals, Dr. Z.'s complicated trajectory leaves her well positioned to reflect insightfully on the core concern in our study: the complex and variable role of culture as growing hyperdiversity presents American clinicians, health-care institutions, and the culture of biomedicine itself with new challenges and dilemmas. Her recollections and insights reflect a wide variety of salient personal and professional experiences. These include a difficult personal and familial experience of immigration, a challenging process of professional retraining, and a fitful process of socialization into a rapidly changing medical subspecialty (subculture). Equally important are her ongoing clinical efforts to bridge cultural divides between herself and her patients, her attempts to leverage her own cultural background in a manner that will enhance her capacities to diagnose and treat her patients, and her efforts to avoid falling into the trap of assuming that a cultural "match" inevitably will yield clinical benefit.

In a sense, Dr. Z. epitomizes hyperdiversity in action. An immigrant physician, Dr. Z.'s cultural background and linguistic skills work to her advantage in some clinical encounters, work against her in others, and make little difference in still others. Despite her keen sensitivity to the importance of seeing the person behind the patient, she is prone to frustration when treating an immigrant patient with whom she shares no common language. She is ready to work with interpreters—whether live and in the flesh or accessible via computerized communication device—but will admit that such interventions are likely to disrupt her work and make her "work life more difficult." She can easily recall instances in which her background helped avoid misdiagnosis of a Russian-speaking patient, or helped a clinical team understand how cultural context might explain the "annoying" conduct of a relative more familiar with the Soviet medical system than the American. Yet she can just as easily recount instances in which cultural familiarity impeded her work. Through sensitivity, optimism, and willingness to take on a leadership role in shaping her clinical environment, Dr. Z. and clinicians like her have the capacity to offer thoughtful responses to the thorny dilemmas associated with the practice of biomedicine in today's hyperdiverse United States.

Note

1. One way to relieve Dr. Z.'s (and, presumably, her colleagues') sense that non-English-speaking patients will inevitably pose a burden might involve

administrative streamlining; if clinical and interpretive services could be efficiently coordinated, then interpreter consultations might be able to take place without adding a great deal of time to the clinical interaction. Another potential step, addressed in some detail by the interpreters we interviewed, might involve workshops for clinicians to help them understand the interpreter's role and communicate effectively within interpreted interactions (see chapter 3, this volume).

References

Kleinman, Arthur. 1988. *The Illness Narratives: Suffering, Healing, and the Human Condition.* New York: Basic Books.

Kleinman, Arthur, and Peter Benson. 2006. "Anthropology in the Clinic: The Problem of Cultural Competency and How to Fix It." *PLoS Medicine* 3(10): e294. Available at: http://www.plosmedicine.org/article/info%3Adoi%2F10.1371%2Fjournal.pmed.0030294 (accessed June 24, 2011).

Lakes, Kimberly, Steven R. López, and Linda C. Garro. 2006. "Cultural Competence and Psychotherapy: Applying Anthropologically Informed Conceptions of Culture." *Psychotherapy: Theory, Research, Practice, and Training* 43(4): 380–96.

Luhrmann, Tanya M. 2000. *Of Two Minds: An Anthropologist Looks at American Psychiatry.* New York: Vintage Books.

Chapter 7

Psychiatry in a Flat World

SADEQ RAHIMI, SETH DONAL HANNAH,
AND MARY-JO DELVECCHIO GOOD

My worry personally is—being a leader in the field—is the disappearance of thoughtfulness regarding issues of culture and the importance of
making a relationship with the patient.
—Psychiatrist and director of an academic medical center

ACCORDING to Clive Unsworth, the Golden Age of psychiatry as a
profession started in the late nineteenth century and continued
through the twentieth, but never made it to the twenty-first
(1991, 1993). Yet in recent years, startling advances in neuroscience and
psychopharmacology have given psychiatrists powerful new tools with
potential to improve the lives of patients with psychiatric disorders.
Despite these advances, the profession is challenged by a growing "disparities" movement pushing for psychiatry to be more responsive to the
needs of diverse racial, ethnic, cultural, religious, and socioeconomic
groups and to reduce barriers to access and care (Smedley, Stith, and
Nelson 2003; Good et al. 2003; Chang 2003; Metzl 2009). In addition, various groups participating in the anti-psychiatry movement, which has
its roots in the 1960s and 1970s, continue to question the very efficacy of
modern psychiatric treatments (Szasz 1961, 1970; Laing 1969).

These new as well as older challenges raise fundamental questions
about the current state of psychiatric practice. How are these challenges
experienced by psychiatric clinicians practicing today? Is psychiatry experiencing a renewed period of openness and engagement with forces outside of medicine, or is it mired in a self-contained culture of psychiatry,
with a coherent set of guiding principles and practices? In this chapter,

we examine these questions through a series of interviews conducted with high-level psychiatric clinicians and directors at academic medical centers in Greater Boston. We find that these clinicians are practicing in an increasingly flat world where their professional dominance is challenged by a much more open social environment, in part a result of global flows of knowledge, due to scientific innovations such as the Internet, and global flows of people, due to increased immigration and demographic shifts. These forces complicate how clinicians define and fulfill their core mission.

Clinicians we interviewed were called to deliver good-quality biomedical psychiatry, good-quality psychotherapy, as well as good-quality culturally sensitive care, all in an environment of budget austerity, exploding hyperdiversity, and the constraints of managed care and quality assurance organizations. For the clinicians we interviewed, it was the engagement with these social, political, and institutional forces that constituted their contemporary culture of psychiatry.

Evolving Conceptualizations of the Culture of Psychiatry

Contemporary debates about ways to think about the culture of psychiatry have been characterized by critiques that often treat psychiatry as a coherent, closed, self-sustaining entity, defined largely by its practitioners. During the anti-psychiatry movement of the late 1960s, Thomas Szasz, R. D. Laing, and others denounced psychiatry's seemingly purposive confounding of deviance and disease, social control and healing, or institutional power and humane treatment (Szasz 1961, 1970; Laing 1969). Though sophistications in community-based care and psychopharmacology calmed much of the early anti-psychiatry rhetoric, voices of critique are still alive today. One of the most prominent contemporary critics is Peter Breggin, a Harvard and Case Western University–educated psychiatrist, whose books speak volumes to his disdain for contemporary psychiatry's dependence on psychopharmacology: *Toxic Psychiatry* (1991), *Talking Back to Prozac* (1994), *Talking Back to Ritalin* (2001), and *Brain-Disabling Treatments in Psychiatry* (1997). Although Breggin strives to reform rather than dismiss psychiatry, others argue for its abolishment as a medical specialty and claim "psychiatric drugs are worthless, and most of them are harmful . . . and are dangers to your health" (Stevens 2001, 2002).

On the other side of the debate, proponents characterize psychiatry as contributing to a social good. As William Carpenter asserts in an editorial in the *American Journal of Psychiatry*, "Society has a moral responsibility for its sick and disabled citizens. Psychiatry assumes this responsibility when clinicians provide care and treatment to mentally ill patients, many of whom suffer from the worst diseases afflicting humans" (1999, 1307).

Carpenter argues that psychiatrists have the moral authority of recognizing what is right for their patients above and beyond the patients' own understanding, asserting that patients "often lack insight into the nature of their afflictions, their causes, and their need for treatment" (1307).

Another conceptualization of psychiatry as an entity manifesting its own culture is developed by the anthropologist Tanya Luhrmann in her study of a major psychiatric center (2000). *Of Two Minds* documents how psychiatry operates in her research setting with one faction proudly promoting a disease model grounded in the biomedical sciences and the other faction promoting a psychodynamic model focusing on the unconscious. Luhrmann views psychiatry as holding these competing and complementary paradigms simultaneously, with different professions and different individuals within a profession associated with one stance or the other, thus giving psychiatry its particular culture.

Although these conceptualizations of psychiatry capture some important aspects of psychiatric practice, they both conceive a closed view of culture that does not fully allow for local variation in psychiatric practice in response to factors external to the discipline (for similar critiques of the closed nature of organizations, see Good 1995; Hahn and Gaines 1985; see also Powell and Dimaggio 1991). As a result, these formulations do not adequately capture the most salient aspects of contemporary psychiatric practice. Psychiatry should not be seen solely as suffering from a case of double-mindedness, but as a cosmopolitan profession, defined by globalizing standards and knowledge and local forms of practice (Good 1995).

Culture and Psychiatry

"The problem with culture," wrote the literary theorist Stephen Greenblatt, is that "it is impossibly vague and encompassing, and the few things that seem excluded . . . are almost immediately reincorporated in the actual use of the word" (1990, 225). As an alternative paradigm in approaching the questions traditionally addressed through the notion of "culture," Greenblatt suggests conceptualizing the idea through attention to opposite forces simultaneously pushing and pulling. A closer examination of the concept of culture indicates it "gestures to what appear to be opposite things: constraint and mobility" (1990, 225). The advantage offered by using Greenblatt's framing of the cultural paradigm is that it addresses the relational dynamics and effects of a specific social setting, instead of attempting to capture a static snapshot or essence of a system.

Other theorists also attend to the relational dynamics and oppositional tensions within institutions, including that of psychiatry (for example, Bakhtin 1994; Even-Zohar 1990; Minh-Ha 1995; Voloshinov 1986; Good and Hannah 2010; Hahn and Gaines 1985). In "Cultural Studies of

Biomedicine," Mary-Jo DelVecchio Good argues that cultural studies of contemporary biomedicine should focus on the dynamic relationship between local and international worlds of knowledge, technology, and practice (1995, 461).

According to Good, the practice of medicine, including psychiatry, is characterized by cultural traffic between international centers of bio-medicine and the local contexts in which medical care is provided to patients. Internationalism in the production of biotechnologies—from pharmaceuticals to medically engineered machinery for imagining and monitoring the body and the brain—influences local cultures of clinical practice as standards of care are altered and the bioscience underpin-nings of clinical narratives become increasingly transformed. The com-plexities, and messiness, of these social interchanges produce the culture of clinical practice (Good 1995, 470–71).

The conceptualizations of the culture of psychiatry and of medicine asserted by Greenblatt (push and pull) and Good (global cultural traffic) call our attention to the deep social embeddedness of organizations, the professions, and medical knowledge. As Jonathan Metzl's book *The Protest Psychosis* (2009) shows, what can be seen as universal psychi-atric disorders—schizophrenia in this case—are in fact intimately tied to social norms such as changing gender roles and racism. Moreover, as Good and Seth Hannah note, "Medical cultures are socially constructed worlds of illness and healing that vary across local and national con-texts. They stem from the dynamic relationship between the local and global worlds of the production of knowledge, technologies, markets and clinical standards" (2010, 458).

In the rest of this chapter, we examine how clinicians and support staff in our study experience the practice of modern psychiatry. We find that, as Greenblatt and Good suggest, their experience is significantly influenced by global flows of knowledge, global flows of people, and the political, institutional and social environments in which they practice. We discuss these three themes in turn.

Psychiatry and a Flat World: Global Flows of Knowledge

Our interviews with clinicians and support staff in greater Boston revealed the myriad ways the social and institutional environment shapes contemporary psychiatric practice. We began with open-ended questions about the role of culture, however defined, in psychiatry. In many responses, the answers associated the role of culture in psychiatry with wider phenomena in the world. For example, a senior psychiatrist and director working in a major teaching hospital spoke about the impact that globalization is having on contemporary practice of psychiatry.

Q: Your thoughts on how culture influences the practice of psychiatry . . . In short, does culture matter in the practice of psychiatry?

Director: A few things come to my mind, the first of which is the word *globalization,* which has something to do with the world becoming flat. With access to knowledge and services growing, I think again because of the Internet, which is as revolutionary as the printing press or more so, that affects everything. It certainly affects psychiatry and the practice of medicine in general.

It is worth noting that this excerpt is from the very opening of the interview. The interviewee is responding to our first question, which simply asked whether culture matters to psychiatry. From the point of view of this director, the very first response and association for the question "Does culture matter to psychiatry?" is "Yes, the world is becoming flat." By claiming that expanding access to knowledge and psychiatric services around the world is having a major affect on psychiatry, he explicitly relates the practice of psychiatry to the wider influences of the social world.

The idea of the world becoming flat is an allusion to Thomas Friedman and his theories of the fundamental change that our civilization is going through (2005). According to Friedman, these changes are due in large part to new technologies and to new social and economic relations born of those new technologies. Friedman captures the broad sense of this change through the metaphor of a world that is becoming flat, in which traditional topologies of power and modes of hierarchical structuring no longer hold.

The director also goes directly to the notion of a revolution that is due to scientific innovations and what may be termed the *democratization* of knowledge as engendered by the Internet. But the director also focuses on the flatness embodied by the global expansion of access to psychiatric treatment, and the global expansion of psychiatric epidemiology. He argues that many of the core elements of psychiatry, such as the belief in the universal, biological basis of psychiatric disorders, are challenged as the practice of psychiatry and psychiatric epidemiology spreads around the globe:

If psychiatry is about how individuals operate, and how the individual brain operates, and if human brains are designed or evolved, if you will, to operate in tribal groups, and not as individuals but in groups, which were families and extended families, and then villages, and cities, and then nations, then how the brain adapts, both within itself, which have to do with genetics and axis one diagnoses and problems . . . differences may exist in the genetic manifestation of psychiatric diagnoses, about which we're learning more.

The director is pointing out that psychiatry, which in his view is about how an individual's brain operates, does not function autonomously; it is embedded within layers of social context expanding from families to nations. As a result, the biological foundation of psychiatric diagnosis may differ as the brain adapts across these social contexts. With the rise of global psychiatry and psychiatric epidemiology, it is possible to empirically measure this proposition. The director makes note of this:

> Well, psychiatry itself, human brains are what human brains are and have always been, although there are some interesting statistics that are showing maybe depression is rising. Why would depression be rising absolutely, if the research is to be believed? Well it's pretty interesting. One might suggest that it's related to global phenomenon, more alienation.

The director is recognizing that the foundational claim of modern biomedical psychiatry—the universality of the brain as the basis of psychiatric disorder—is seriously challenged by globalization and the flatness of the world as embodied by global psychiatry. If depression, for example, were merely a function of biology, why would its prevalence be rising over time around the world?

The director suggests that it may be related to another global phenomenon, "more alienation." Building on his earlier point that individual brains are embedded in various levels of social context, he argues that because individual brains "respond to stressors in different ways," the increased immigration and mixing of heterogeneous groups associated with globalization may lead to alienation as individuals travel through different social milieus:

> Brains and whatever their genetic endowment might be operate collectively within a family, but more importantly that family or family group is a manifestation of the larger culture, even new cultures. An Italian and an Irishman, that's a new kind of family culture. But those are families or individuals that operate within their social milieu. So an Irish family may be different from another Irish family, but they may be in Ireland. But an Irish family coming to an Italian city—and those are just European—has a new challenge.

Here, he gives the example of an individual in an Irish family who may be stable living within their own social milieu, but will face a challenge as they move into a new one. This is because of the way the brain must adapt to stressors in the new environment, the director continues:

> As immigration and globalization and heterogeneous groups are happening, it's a challenge. Within an individual brain, which responds to stressors in different ways, and we know that now increasingly genetically, and if you believe that it is a stressor to travel, it is a stressor to be

> alien, then that can impact on the manifestation of the diathesis or pre-disposition for the manifestation of psychiatric disorders. So what mitigates stress? I think what mitigates stress is the comfort that comes, or safety, I guess you would say, from having your roots in a familiar—which has in its root family—in a familiar environment. So the safety with your family is there, and as it's not available, the stress is more, and as the stress is more, the manifestation of psychiatric illnesses is more.

According to the director, the newly flat world implies a series of social stressors that shape the expression of psychiatric illness as the biology of the brain interacts with changes in the social environment. This provides one possible explanation for increasing global rates of depression, as increased global migration increases stress and alienation.

The significant point is that the global flows of knowledge associated with the globalization of psychiatry have had a dramatic impact on the way this director views psychiatry and how he and other clinicians we interviewed experience psychiatric practice. This supports the idea that there is no closed, coherent, self-sustaining culture of psychiatry; it is heavily influenced by the larger social world, especially trends associated with the newly globalized world.

Global Flows of People:
How Clinicians Respond

The social embeddedness of psychiatry is also revealed in the ways psychiatrists interact with their patients. This is especially relevant today, as immigration and demographic shifts bring hyperdiversity to patient populations and the discipline of psychiatry. Clinicians we interviewed argued that the social and cultural experiences of their patients are critical to the formation and expression of psychiatric illness, and must be discovered and considered if excellent care is to be provided. Although each clinician tended to have a unique approach, the process of discovering and accounting for cultural and social difference generally involved the issues of power, knowledge, and face validity.

The notion of knowledge and its association with power as a significant feature of the "psy" institution, as Foucault would put it, were implicitly embedded in the responses given by the psychiatrist director we just discussed. Throughout many of our interviews, however, the same sentiment was far more explicitly stated. In the following excerpt, the relationship between knowledge and power is clearly spelled out. While discussing the diversity committee at his hospital and the training sessions the security guards organize in response to the different ethnicities and cultural groups represented in the patient and staff populations of the hospital, we had the following exchange:

Q: Does culture help you in any way?

Security Guard: Sure, it would. I think it would just, gives you, empowers you. You know, knowledge is power, and it gives you more knowledge to do your job more effectively and to create a safer environment for everybody, and to make your patients happier. [Nervous laughter] You know, a happy patient is not going to act out on you. [Laughs again] We like to make them comfortable, to let them know that you're aware, that you're sensitive to them.

Part of the reason the security guard's comments engage the questions of power and control in such strikingly explicit terms is that he is directly charged with ensuring order within the psychiatric environment. He took special care to point out how proud he was of his understanding that knowledge is truly important in this environment, if one is to keep the patients from disorderly behavior.

Now let us compare the security guard's remarks with those of the psychiatrist director, as he responded to the same question.

Q: Is the issue of culture helpful in any way?

Director: Culture can't be defined by race and ethnicity, country of origin. It can be defined by religious and spiritual beliefs, and socioeconomic status, what have you. So the more sensitivity one has, the more a physician is going to be able to identify those things that might mitigate the stress and also might accelerate the doctor-patient connection. So when I was in Palm Beach a couple of weeks ago, the approach I'm going to make, what I'm going to wear, the words I choose to use, the metaphor, which is an important part of relating to whatever the patient might be, becomes important. . . . If I'm dealing with the Palm Beach group, I might be talking with metaphors that are about golf courses and clubs and about how hard it is to deal with all that money you have. That's an awareness that, as a clinician, I can make a connection. So that I have face validity as a person who can recognize the person that I'm speaking with. Make a connection. So as the cultures are globalizing, it's only happening more and more.

What this clinician is expressing implicitly is not at all dissimilar to what the security guard conveyed in more explicit terms earlier. A sense of cultural familiarity is deemed important here because it gives the clinician *face validity* as a person who recognizes the person he is speaking with. Recognition of the patient, a capacity to name or locate the world of that patient, in other words, is suggested here as the evidence patients use to attribute knowledge to the clinician. What is tacitly embedded in the logical structure of this excerpt is that it is the face validity of the clinician which is at stake in the clinical encounter, and the ability to recognize the patient is vital to the patient's granting such face validity or trust (and the power and authority that accompanies it) to the clinician. The power, in other words, is granted in the form of deference and trust; and it is granted in response to the clinician's demonstration of his ability to masterfully comport himself according to a specific code of knowledge or face validity.

What emerges out of the examination of this logic is fundamentally similar to the idea expressed by the security guard about the importance of knowledge as a form of power. They both consider cultural knowledge important in successfully engaging with psychiatric patients. However, while the security guard speaks in broad terms about different cultural groups and ethnicities, the director speaks of the particular cultural orientations of individuals or smaller, non-ethnically based social groups. In this case, wealthy golfers in Palm Beach, Florida, have a distinct culture, but not one that is likely to be addressed by diversity committees and special hospital-wide celebrations.

In another example, the director speaks of the need to determine a woman's religious belief before counseling her about her family planning options:

> A clinician was presenting the case of a young woman who was not engaged to her boyfriend, but she was pregnant, and they had just broken up. I listened to the presentation of the case, and the first question I asked, which the clinician had not asked of this person who was now pregnant, and pregnant only six weeks, and so I asked, "Is she Catholic?" And the clinician was a little puzzled by this. That was the first question that came to mind for me in this situation as a critical element, based on my experience and sensitivity to that, which obviously the clinician did not have, which is, "I can't go further with any advice without knowing that." Without understanding the socioeconomic status, the employment status, the cultural status, I ask often, "Is this the first person that's been to college in their family history?" So all of the aspects that make up who an individual is is required, I believe, to make the connection with that individual, and then to understand how that individual is operating within that social sphere.

In this way, the director's comments resonate with Elizabeth Carpenter-Song's focus on recognition in the formation of clinical relationships in chapter 8 of this volume. He does not approach his patients with the culturally reductive stance of "I know you," he seeks to elicit more information, instead asking, "Who are you?"

The comments from the security guard and director underscore the complexity of power relations as the social topology changes with global and regional flows of knowledge and people. As a result of these global flows, and the interaction they necessitate between clinicians and patients with different cultural orientations, to be granted power by the patient, clinicians need to impress the patient by telling him or her that, in effect, "I may not know you personally, yet my knowledge allows me to categorically recognize you." Once the significance of the patient's bestowing of power to the psychiatrist becomes evident, it is easy to see how global flows of knowledge and people can complicate and even excite the traditional medical establishment.

The Institutional Environment

The clinicians we spoke with revealed that, in their experience, contemporary psychiatric practice is characterized by an open culture influenced by a variety of factors external to its disciplinary imperatives. Although the experiences and perspectives discussed earlier focused on the new flatness of the world as characterized by global flows of knowledge and people, other clinicians focused on more local constraints on their professional autonomy and modes of practice.

One frequently mentioned factor is the current environment of budget austerity and the at times overwhelming demand for efficiency concurrent with overwhelming demand for services. Some clinicians worry about their financial viability, whereas directors and managers worry about changes in their practice style that austerity and efficiency necessitate. The psychiatrist director discussed in the last section captured this feeling well:

> I don't think it is being experienced as an anxiety except by the leaders. . . . Psychiatrists in the field are so damn busy and the demand for their services is so much that the only thing they are anxious about is to see if they're going to be able to keep making a living. The leaders, the thought leaders in the fields, however, may be wondering . . . My worry personally is, being a leader in the field, is the disappearance of thoughtfulness regarding issues of culture and the importance of making a relationship with the patient.

The anxiety over the future of psychiatry and its identity is expressed in other terms, that of worrying about the loss of a certain relationship with the patient. It is possible to recognize in this comment, a more pervasive or existential sense of threat behind the intellectual concern about the relationship with patients.

Other clinicians are so busy with the exigencies of clinical care and the time pressures of productivity targets that they are unable to engage in other priorities, such as research. A psychologist director of a community mental health service spoke to us at length about the high demand for services in her clinic, and the productivity management system she enacts in response to her tight budgets. She described how these factors shape her clinical practice:

> Those of us who are attracted to this kind of work tend to be more in the bent of a clinician, not a research thinker, and not that you can't do both, but when you are so heavily laden in the direct clinical work, and you got a patient that's trying to kill themselves, or you got a patient that is—I had a drunken woman asleep on my floor the other day. When you're caught up with that, it's very hard to take that luxury—and that is the word to use—to step back and, you really have to shift your thinking ever so slightly, think about it in a measured way.

These external forces are also shaping the experiences of nurses who work in psychiatric settings. A nurse who works in the same academic medical center as the psychiatrist director and security guard discussed in the previous section has several decades of clinical experience in that hospital, and has witnessed dramatic changes in the way psychiatry has been practiced over time. She recounted the story of how the ward she worked on had changed over time both physically, as it moved from one building to another, and culturally, in the sense that it used to be an open unit and is now a closed one.

According to her account, however, the change was much larger than either of those. In her opinion, psychiatry has undergone a change over the past few decades that reflects larger social and economic realities. These include changing patient demographics, changes in the political economy of medicine, and changes in the dominant modes of psychiatric practice. Regarding changes on the unit in response to changing demographics, she observed,

> On the voluntary unit, we would often not admit people who couldn't speak much English, because you couldn't participate in the groups, you couldn't participate in the therapy if we couldn't talk to them. We would sort of say, "Well, they're not really appropriate for us, how can they participate?" [Then] we came over here [to the new facility], and now we totally don't turn anybody away anymore. We use interpreters, and have figured out ways to treat people, you know, the doctors are always interviewing them with interpreters. We use people that speak Spanish whether it's, you know, nurses, doctors, or cleaning people we'll use. They're excellent. . . . So it has changed, it's much more all-inclusive, and we're much more figuring out a way to treat anybody from any culture.

The hospital has evolved, this nurse says, to accommodate the language needs of their increasingly diverse patients by adding interpreter services that have become more sophisticated over time and hiring more diverse staff, particularly cleaning and lower-level administrative staff, who can help facilitate the participation of new patients.

At the same time, the hospital has had to respond to demographic change, it was experiencing wider changes in the political economy of medicine and the practice of psychiatry that have prioritized biomedical intervention, acute stabilization, and short-term treatment. The nurse explained it this way:

> We don't do as much therapy, we're not trying to, you know, behaviorally change people that much, maybe a tiny bit, and we're not trying to delve into people's, uh, trying to really psychiatrically do, you know, therapy and long-term *psycho-surgery*.[1] We're much more trying to get a person so that they can go back out.

Interestingly, she considers the move toward shorter term, rehabilitation-style treatment makes it easier to cope with cultural and linguistic difference. If you're not focused on long-term talk-based therapy, in her opinion, being able to speak the patient's language (and by extension, using cultural knowledge to make a therapeutic interpersonal connection) is less necessary. As the nurse says, acute psychiatric rehabilitation is

> easier to do when even no matter what language, what culture you are, when we can just kind of deal with maybe medicines or ECT and that kind of thing, and get a person better . . . The questions that we ask are things like: Are you sleeping? How's your interest? Are you hearing voices? That kind of thing. So they're all much more concrete. So we've lost some of the therapy part, or, but that happened to everybody here, so it has made it easier to treat all kinds of people.

Interestingly, the nurse is claiming that the rise of biomedical psychiatry makes the cultural issues less relevant and treatment in general more productive. When we asked her if this were the case, she responded,

> In some ways, yes, more efficient. It's like [snaps her fingers to indicate swiftness and efficiency], chop, chop, and "See you later" [laughs]. . . . It's very, you know, it's trying to cut health care costs. We don't keep people as long. We used to take people off of their antidepressants completely, and then give them ECT, and then start them back up on these antidepressants for three or four weeks and then discharge them. Now we let them stay on their antidepressants, we start ECT right away, they've already been on their antidepressants, and we barely give them a day or so. They can even get ECT that morning and go home. . . . It's much more efficient, much more timely, 'cause insurance companies don't wanna pay, and the cost of being in the hospital is so much more.

As Luhrmann describes in discussing the two approaches to psychiatry, the biomedical and the psychodynamic, the changes experienced by this nurse, and others who practice at her academic medical center, raise a series of questions about what is gained and what is lost in this process of change. According to the psychiatric director we interviewed, the flatness of globalization necessitates a deeper attention to how individual brains interact with the social world, requiring additional time and attention spent on developing relationships and connections with patients. Meanwhile, the nurse calls attention to other powerful forces that can improve the lives of patients without engaging in social and cultural relationships. This is no easy task, and as Luhrmann says in closing, "We are so tempted to see ourselves as fixable, perfectible brains. But the loss of our souls is a high price to pay" (2000, 293). On the one hand, people from various groups can now come in, be accepted, and get their treatment with hardly any significant obstacles standing between them and the care they need. At the same time, it is hard to receive care without losing close and meaningful personal contact.

The nurse's comments are specifically significant in that they speak of changes in psychiatry in a way that captures both the inevitability of the process and the sense of ambivalence that runs through that process. She captures the complexity of change in her intimate account. One difference between the comments of this nurse and those of psychiatrists is the orientation of the anxiety, rather than its presence or absence. Whereas directors typically spoke of the future of psychiatry as a professional identity and a career path, the nurse and clinicians often spoke of anxiety in reference to the quality of care that they were able to deliver to their patients. What remained constant across all these narratives, however, was that the fundamentals of the profession had changed in relation to social and institutional forces and that the evaluation and consequences of that change were still unclear.

The discussion has brought us back to the points with which we started the chapter. We have discussed the notion of change in the context of psychiatry as a personal career and an institutional identity, along with the implicit and explicit anxieties that can accompany that change. One point that has been driven home repeatedly in our interviews is that psychiatry is not a monolithic structure with an a priori or even specific identity. It is important, in other words, to keep in mind that psychiatry changes gradually but concretely and constantly, that it has a complex and emergent identity or culture, that it is not in any way separate from the society that contains it, and that we should therefore avoid the temptation of trapping it in such convenient conceptual models.

Conclusion

To further underscore the openness of contemporary psychiatric practice, we conclude with comments from a psychiatrist director at an academic medical center, quoted previously. Whereas the nurse viewed the hospital as making strides toward seriously expanding services to individuals with diverse cultural and linguistic needs, the director viewed these changes as severely inadequate and hampered by a variety of forces. When the director told us that both changes, which he described in positive terms such as increasing sophistication and inclusiveness, were coming too slowly to the hospital in which he worked, we asked him what obstacles slowed them down. In response, he listed four items:

- "The size of the institution. It's too big to change quickly . . . practically, it takes a long time to change things."
- "It is an inherently conservative hospital. They don't do new crazy things. Crazy things, whatever, like cross-cultural shit."
- "The communities that it has historically served in the neighborhood have been white working class . . . the demand for local, by local people for local treatments hasn't been culturally or race-based."
- "It was a very racist, very segregated . . . it wasn't until World War II that even Jewish residents were accepted here for residency. The most diverse thing you could be here was Catholic."

Despite their diversity, all four items point toward a single conclusion: the systemic embeddedness of psychiatry and its culture within the larger social context. Each item is located within an outwardly expanding set of overlapping concentric spheres, with psychiatry operating within and across their boundaries. Item one represents the center of four circles referring to the physical features of institution itself. Item two references the institution's larger culture and history. Item three leads outside the institution to its local physical and social surroundings. And item four connects the institution and its surrounding community to the society at large, and with the long traditions of racism and segregation.

The director's enumeration of these obstacles beautifully portrays the complex cultural traffic between multiple levels of social organization. By describing the factors that constrain his ability to reform his practice in the direction of sophistication and inclusiveness, he reveals an essential truth about the modern practice of psychiatry. No longer are the modalities of care strictly determined by the internal logic of psychiatric theory, training, and practice—as maintained and promoted within the discipline itself or its visionary "thought leaders." Psychiatrists today are forced to confront a newly flat world, where their day-to-day work is shaped by broader influences from the social, political, and institutional environment.

We recognize that the core aspects of contemporary psychiatric practice are not, and have likely never been, determined solely by internal debates and actions of the profession itself, its theoretical foundation, or its evidence base. However, the data presented in this chapter shows that psychiatry is increasingly open to global flows of knowledge and people, each with their own cultural characteristics and imperatives, and this flatness challenges the notion of a coherent culture of psychiatry that operates as an independent actor.

But the flatness of globalization has a flip side; it is not only that ideas and people are more interconnected than ever "out there" in the world, but also that these global influences are ending up on our own doorstep in the wake of increased immigration and the diversity of ideas and individuals here at home. As our interviews show, the culture of psychiatry is now subject to these influences as well, especially considering the hyperdiverse clinical settings in which many clinicians now work and the hyperdiversity among the clinicians themselves. These global influences cannot help but reshape local forms of practice in psychiatry.

With this flatness in mind, instead of talking about the culture of psychiatry as a single, internally coherent, agency-bearing medical specialty— perhaps we need to be speaking about, and conducting further empirical investigations of, the different pushes and pulls and forms of global cultural traffic we argue are the true elements of the culture of psychiatry. Such an approach allows the consideration of social factors such as race, ethnicity, social class, or religion alongside institutional factors such as organizational culture and political economy, both under the rubric of cultural analysis.

Note

1. The term *psycho-surgery* is used here to characterize the biomechanism of psychotherapy, not lobotomy.

References

Bakhtin, Mikhail. 1994. "Social Heteroglossia." In *The Bakhtin Reader: Selected Readings of Bakhtin, Medvedev, Voloshinov,* edited by Pam Morris. London: Edward Arnold.

Breggin, Peter. 1991. *Toxic Psychiatry.* New York: St. Martin's Press.

———. 1994. *Talking Back to Prozac.* New York: St. Martin's Press.

———. 1997. *Brain-Disabling Treatments in Psychiatry.* New York: Springer.

———. 2001. *Talking Back to Ritalin.* Cambridge, Mass.: Perseus.

Carpenter, William T., Jr. 1999. "The Challenge to Psychiatry as Society's Agent for Mental Illness Treatment and Research." *American Journal of Psychiatry* 156(9): 1307–10.

Chang, Doris F. 2003. "An Introduction to the Politics of Science: Culture, Race, Ethnicity and the Supplement to the Surgeon General's Report on Mental Health." *Culture, Medicine and Psychiatry* 27(4): 373–83.

Even-Zohar, Itamar. 1990. "Polysystem Studies." Special issue. *Poetics Today* 11(1): 1–268.

Friedman, Thomas L. 2005. *The World Is Flat: A Brief History.* New York: Farrar, Straus and Giroux.

Good, Mary-Jo DelVecchio. 1995. "Cultural Studies of Biomedicine: An Agenda for Research." *Social Science & Medicine* 41(4): 461–73.

Good, Mary-Jo DelVecchio, and Seth Hannah. 2010. "Medical Cultures." In *Handbook of Cultural Sociology*, edited by John R. Hall, Laura Grindstaff, and Ming-Cheng Lo. London: Routledge.

Good, Mary-Jo DelVecchio, Cara James, Byron J. Good, and Anne E. Becker. 2003. "The Culture of Medicine and Racial, Ethnic, and Class Disparities in Healthcare." In *Unequal Treatment: Confronting Racial and Ethnic Disparities in Health Care*, edited by Brian D. Smedley, Adrienne Y. Stith, and Alan R. Nelson. Washington, D.C.: National Academies Press.

Greenblatt, Stephen. 1990. "Culture." In *Critical Terms for Literary Studies*, edited by Frank Lentricchia and Stephen Greenblatt. Chicago: University of Chicago Press.

Hahn, Robert, and Atwood Gaines. 1985. *Physicians of Western Medicine: Anthropological Approaches to Theory and Practice*, vol. v. Boston: Reidel.

Laing, Ronald D. 1969. *The Divided Self*. New York: Random House.

Luhrmann, Tanya M. 2000. *Of Two Minds: The Growing Disorder in American Psychiatry*. New York: Alfred A. Knopf.

Metzl, Jonathan M. 2009. *The Protest Psychosis*. Boston: Beacon Press Books.

Minh-Ha, Trinh. 1995. "No Master Territories." In *The Post-Colonial Studies Reader*, edited by Bill Ashcroft, Gareth Griffiths, and Helen Tiffin. London: Routledge.

Powell, Walter, and Paul DiMaggio. 1991. *The New Institutionalism in Organizational Analysis*. Chicago: University of Chicago Press.

Smedley, Brian D., Adrienne Y. Stith, and Alan Ray Nelson, eds. 2003. *Unequal Treatment: Confronting Racial and Ethnic Disparities in Health Care*. Washington, D.C.: National Academies Press.

Stevens, Lawrence. 2001. "Why Psychiatry Should Be Abolished as a Medical Specialty." Available at: http://www.antipsychiatry.org/abolish.htm (accessed December 1, 2008).

———. 2002. "Psychiatric Drugs: Cure or Quackery?" Available at: http://www.antipsychiatry.org/drugs.htm (accessed December 1, 2008).

Szasz, Thomas. 1961. *The Myth of Mental Illness*. New York: Hoeber-Harper.

———. 1970. *The Manufacture of Madness*. New York: Harper & Row.

Unsworth, Clive. 1991. "Mental Disorder and the Tutelary Relationship: From Pre- to Post-Carceral Legal Order." *Journal of Law and Society* 18(2): 254–78.

———. 1993. "Law and Lunacy in Psychiatry's 'Golden Age'." *Oxford Journal of Legal Studies* 13(4): 479–507.

Voloshinov, V. N. 1986. *Marxism and the Philosophy of Language*. Cambridge, Mass.: Harvard University Press.

Chapter 8

Recognition in Clinical Relationships

ELIZABETH CARPENTER-SONG

A S PREVIOUS chapters in this volume describe in detail, the framing of the study responds to dramatic changes in clinical populations that mirror broad demographic trends toward greater diversity in the population of the United States. In this context, evidence is accumulating that something is deeply wrong in the delivery of health care in the United States, marked particularly by the growing awareness of striking disparities in use and outcomes of health care among minority and low-income populations. Specific to mental health concerns, not only do these populations bear a disproportionate burden of mental illness, they are also less likely to have access to, and receive, needed services; often receive poorer-quality services; and remain underrepresented in mental health research (U.S. Department of HHS 2001; Smedley, Stith, and Nelson 2003).

Medical anthropology is well positioned to engage in documenting structural barriers to access and in offering insight into the local production of disparities through clinical ethnography. As noted in the introduction to this volume, attention to the culture of medicine itself in the production of disparities is a crucial contribution of social studies of medicine (see also Good et al. 2003). Indeed, the critical orientation of medical anthropology provides a firm foundation for homing in on the shortcomings and failures of American medicine. As a discipline, we have trained our gaze on the rifts, breakdowns, and slippages that occur within clinical encounters.

In this vein, concern with the problematic interface between patients and clinicians has deep roots in medical anthropology. Over thirty years of sociolinguistic study of clinical discourse has documented power imbalances in clinician-patient interactions manifesting in the micro-dynamics of what is said and unsaid, who speaks and for how long, who asks questions and interrupts (Fisher and Groce 1990; Mishler 1984; West 1984a, 1984b; West and Frankel 1991). This has led Candace West and Richard Frankel (1991) to characterize the focus of this body of scholarship as one not so much of communication as miscommunication.

These studies have traditionally started from the assumption of a fundamental asymmetry between practitioners and those seeking medical care. Sue Fisher and Stephen Groce characterize the medical interview as a "moment-to-moment battle that mirrors and largely sustains the institutional authority and status of doctors and the reality of genders" (1990, 225). Aaron Cicourel (1983) distinguishes between the "knowledge" of physicians and the "beliefs" of patients (for a critique of notions of belief, see Good 1994). Elliot Mishler (1984) identifies the "two worlds" that collide in the medical encounter as the "voice of medicine" (possessed by physicians) and the "voice of the lifeworld" (expressed by patients). The "voice of the lifeworld" represents the world of everyday life, in which the timing of events and their significance depends upon patients' positioning within the social world. In contrast, the "voice of medicine" represents technical considerations, through which the meaning of events is derived from abstracting and decontextualizing them from particular personal and social contexts (Mishler 1984, 104). The central thrust of Mishler's text is that the ensuing struggle between these two types of worlds fragments and suppresses patients' multifaceted, contextualized, and meaningful accounts.

Mishler's critique echoes the critical stance taken within medical anthropology more generally that has called attention to biomedicine's capacity to erase or ignore the subjective experiences of patients. Ignoring patients' lifeworlds is experienced by patients as a painful and serious threat to their identity, exemplified in Joanne Coyle's analysis of patient dissatisfaction in healthcare in which she found that forty of the forty-one patients interviewed "constructed accounts which showed how their identity had been undermined in some way by the untoward experience. Threats to personal identity included perceptions of being dehumanised, objectified, stereotyped, disempowered, and devalued" (1999, 107).

In the case of chronic illness (to include mental disorders), recasting illness experience as biological pathology entails, in Arthur Kleinman's view, the erasure of the fullness, ambiguity, and particularity of subjective experience such that "something essential to the experience of chronic illness is lost; it is not legitimated as a subject for clinical concern, nor does it receive an intervention" (1988, 6). A similar sense of loss is evidenced in Katherine Young's (1997) Foucauldian ethnography of how biomedicine alienates the self from the body in order that it may become an object accessible to the medical gaze.

In my own experience over the past decade working on various studies that, broadly, examine how individuals and families engage with mental health services in the United States, dissatisfaction and ambivalence have been consistent refrains in people's experience. In my research with families seeking psychiatric services for their children, many parents were highly critical of therapies (Carpenter-Song 2009). An African American father viewed his son's therapy sessions as a "joke." Another African American considered his grandson's counseling "a bunch of hogwash." In a study of adults with serious mental illness, we found that even among individuals who hold highly medicalized views of their problems and agree with the necessity for treatment, many give voice to their disturbing sense that "doctors don't care about people" and "don't treat you like a person" (Carpenter-Song et al. 2010).

What, then, are we to make of happy patients? Many of the patients that my colleagues and I have interviewed in the context of the study describe their clinical relationships in strikingly positive terms. After reading through the consent form, Mary, an African American woman in her mid-eighties, looked at me hesitantly: "Well . . . I'm not sure how helpful I'm going to be. I've had very good care here." When I asked Rick, a fifty-something Euro-American man, to describe an ideal clinician-patient relationship, he chuckled and smiled, "I have it." This sentiment was echoed by Albert, a Euro-American man in his late forties, who described his physician as "the best." Cathy, a sixty-five-year-old Euro-American woman, said about her psychiatrist, "He's an excellent doctor and incredibly ethical so it's easy to trust him. And believe in him. And he's done nothing but good doctoring for eight years. [Laughing] Why not believe in him?! I'd be an idiot not to. . . . Even when I was messed up he didn't go away. [Laughs] So he's a very, very good doctor."

The experiences of these patients challenge us as medical anthropologists. There is not a well-elaborated theoretical framework for approaching positive experiences of Western biomedicine. I would point to the work of Janis Jenkins on experiences of recovery among persons with schizophrenia (Jenkins and Carpenter-Song 2005) and Mary-Jo DelVecchio Good's scholarship on trust and hope (Good et al. 1990, 2003) as fertile ground for consideration of positive dimensions of patient experiences. But, overall, a certain bias in critically oriented medical anthropology reveals itself. Indeed, perhaps our initial reaction to hearing glowing accounts of clinicians is a kind of disbelief or suspicion that the interviewee is being polite or that, as ethnographers, we haven't gotten to the "meat" (or dirt!). Although, as a discipline, we tend to be generously inclined toward non-Western, alternative, and complementary medicines, Western biomedicine is predictably cast in the role of the foil.

However, I certainly would not want this observation to be taken as a call for a suspension of the critical enterprise in medical anthropology.

Nor do I mean to suggest that the trenchant critiques of biomedicine that anthropologists have offered and that I have briefly summarized above are ill placed or that the project of continuing critique is unnecessary. Quite the contrary. In an era of "big business medicine" and "reductionist" approaches to mental health care (Donald 2001), our role as academic watchdogs is all the more crucial. Likewise, this is by no means the experience of all of our participants, particularly those who have been hospitalized involuntarily (for an in-depth consideration of negative aspects of patients' experiences, see chapter 9, this volume).

My point is simply that I think there is much to be learned from positive experiences of engaging in mental health services. For whom are experiences positive or negative? In what contexts? What makes a good clinician? A good patient? Taking positive experiences seriously opens up fresh analytic space for us as researchers to shift from documenting what's wrong toward specifying what may work. In this chapter, I suspend the usual disciplinary focus to explore clinical relationships that are subjectively experienced as positive by patients and clinicians. In so doing, this chapter engages with American psychiatry as a moral enterprise (compare Good 1994). Attention to the on-the-ground realities of clinicians and patients brings forth daily endeavors to negotiate the knife's edge between competence and caring (Good 1995). The reductive potential of biomedicine is well substantiated (and important to critique). But we also want to be aware of—and keep our ears pricked and our eyes open to—the complexity of clinical realities, to include the desires of patients and the motivations of physicians.

This chapter draws on the perspectives and experiences of a diverse group of patients and clinicians. The patients came from diverse racial, ethnic, and class backgrounds. Both women and men gave voice to positive clinical experiences. Patients ranged in age from mid-twenties to mid-eighties. Some had lengthy tenures in mental health services; others were relative newcomers. Likewise, the clinicians considered in this chapter included women and men from diverse racial and ethnic backgrounds.[1] Some clinicians were younger, others older; some were earlier in their careers than others.

In keeping with a central thesis of this volume, I note these characteristics to highlight that there is no easy or obvious way to classify the patients and clinicians in this chapter. This mélange of race, ethnicity, gender, class, and age provides strong support for a characterization of contemporary American medicine as a model of and for hyperdiversity. Furthermore, the diversity of patients and clinicians for whom clinical care is experienced positively points to more universal dimensions of what is desired by patients and the moral register of clinicians' efforts to provide care. In this way, the voices of patients and clinicians may offer a point of entry for the creation of "a more informed universalism" that stands to improve care for all patients.

A Note on Methods

The narrative material examined in this chapter is derived from data collected in phase 2 of the study. In this phase, we conducted semi-structured interviews with patient-clinician dyads[2] to examine experiences of treatment in the context of particular therapeutic relationships as a window into clinical narratives and institutional cultures of care. Patients shared with us their pathways into treatment, the logistics of seeking services, including challenges to obtaining care, and, broadly, their experiences of clinical encounters and reflections on their therapeutic relationships. Clinicians provided insight into the rewards and challenges of working with particular patients as well as reflections on the therapeutic process.

Patient Voices

Rick has been seeing his psychiatrist for about three months, having been referred through a primary care physician when he began experiencing what he describes as acute feelings of depression and anxiety. He was diagnosed with an aggressive form of prostate cancer two years ago and is currently in remission. Rick describes his clinical experience as "part therapy, part exploration." His goal is "to try to understand myself" because "I basically feel that I have limited time." In his account, Rick identified particular communicative and interactive strategies of his psychiatrist that he dubs her "bag of tricks":

> Marriage counseling tips, that's one of the—one of the bag of tricks I guess. Another thing is to—is that um, sometimes when I describe my behavior, like I'll say, I'm, you know, in this—in this thing I'm—I'm impulsive, I'm impulsive about doing this. She'll say, "Well, why is it impulsive?" And—so she kind of sends words back to me that I've used and makes me think about why I use them in describing myself. And that's really helpful.
>
> Another thing is just to let me wander sometimes. But then she can—she'll remember it and bring it back or kind of—I guess this is what's good about therapy—she can relate it to something else I said either earlier that session or in a previous session.
>
> Another thing she does is handles the silences well. Um, I mean I'm not someone who clams up, but sometimes after gettin' it out, you know, I'm quiet for a little bit and she's—she goes with that for what I think is just the right amount, you know, she'll—she'll be quiet with me. She'll let me be quiet and then gently say something—maybe ask me what I'm thinking or where I'm going with it. And, it's great. Yeah.

Cathy has been in the mental health system since the mid-1960s, when she was institutionalized in a state hospital for four years. Cathy described horrifying experiences of care over the years—therapists "who wanted me to be their therapist," a psychologist who forced himself on her, and physicians who did not take her medical complaints seriously on account of her mental illness. She has been seeing her current psychiatrist for eight years, a man she affectionately refers to as, "The Famous Dr. B." and describes as "consistent" and "available" and—tongue-in-cheek—as a "high-functioning doctor!" She describes what Dr. B. is able to accomplish even in a very limited amount of time: "You'd be surprised how much good he can pack in to fifteen or twenty minutes. Not just the medicine— he keeps up with what's happening on a daily, weekly, and monthly basis in that fifteen, twenty minutes—how my relationships are going, how my environment's going, if I'm safe. You know, um—progress, um—negative progress. All kinds of things."

For Cathy, the "best thing" about receiving care at this clinic is the "flexibility" and that "I get to be an adult and the primary person in my own care."

Albert has been receiving comprehensive medical and mental health care for nineteen years following neurosurgery to remove a brain tumor. His surgeon at the time was recommended "on the basis of personality" by the chief of surgery: "He thought we'd get along." In the wake of developing epilepsy following the surgery—Albert attributes this directly to the surgeon's inexperience and incompetence—he now views the reasoning behind selecting this physician as "horrendous" and "obscene." Shaking his head, he fixed his gaze on me: "Can you imagine?" The clinicians that Albert has seen since stand in stark contrast to his experience of entering the health-care system. Describing his current neurologist, Albert stated, "If he told me to jump off a cliff I'd be a little surprised, but if he said so, I would." As part of his "comprehensive" care, Albert has been seeing a therapist since his first brain surgery. Though he has changed mental health providers over the years, he views these professionals as "part of the apparatus" of an institution that he has come to consider his "home base." Echoing others in the study, Albert views his interactions with the social worker as "one of the few opportunities you get to tell somebody what's bothering you where they don't fight back."

Mary has been seeing her psychiatrist for the past six years, having been referred by her primary care physician, who told her, "Maybe you have anxiety." Mary describes herself as an "extremely busy person." She currently serves on the board of her church, was president of the local chapter of Habitat for Humanity for four years, and continues to work full time. Although she is, in her words, "up in age," Mary is usually at home in the evenings only one night per week. Before seeking care, she was "feeling drained" and was having difficulty sleeping. Her experiences in the mental health unit have been very positive and she contrasts this with her experiences in the emergency department of the same hospital, where she has recently endured waits as long as sixteen hours. She described being able to tell "right away" that her psychiatrist was a caring person, someone who "spoke with a gentle manner." In this narrative passage, she elaborates the high stakes of good clinical relationships:

> Right away, I knew he was a person that cared about me. And I told him I didn't like taking pills or a lot of medicine and he found something that he thought would be appropriate for my situation and I had, you know, a large, a great number of conversations with him over time about my life and, uh, he would give me some advice, you know, on what, you know, not so much advice—his opinion. And I valued it because he was—it was right and I applied it and so, I don't get the anxiety as often. I still— you know, and I wasn't sleeping. I had lost about eighteen nights of sleep. I was worn out, so. He, uh, he's a very, uh, I think he's one of those people that you feel something chest to chest, breast to breast when you talk with him and he's, um, he's a real—I said I can't move outta Boston or I'll lose [my doctor]! [Laughs] I have to stay here for that! But my experience in, in the behavioral neurology has been very positive and um, I just wish that most doctors were as sensitive to the needs of their patients as he was and as caring and I think part of your recovery is related to your psychological thinking—you, you trust that person, you know they're telling you what's right and you believe in them. I think that's part of your recovery along with the medicine.

Clinician Voices

Reflecting on the therapeutic process, the clinicians in the study have described the conditions they view as central to good care. Dr. Ruiz, a psychiatrist, approaches the clinical encounter as a learning process and emphasized that it is the patient who is positioned to educate the clinician: "I don't like the word *psychoeducation* very much because it implies that I have some truth that they [patients] do not know and that I have to educate them about that."

Dr. Ruiz spoke at length about the importance of forging a connection with his patients:

> So for me it is first of all, what brings the patient to me? How can I connect with the person? . . . So for me the major issue is how to make that connection with the person [pause] how to kind of, there is confluence in that. And from there, I feel that from there, everything is, you know, a given. Because then I can show the patient, okay, listen. I have taken seriously what you're saying and can I show you this other [way] and the person opens up and says okay, well show me! What else? When they know—when you know that you know that there is a situation where the

patients say, "Oh, so you get—you get what I'm saying, right. You get what I'm saying!" And the moment that the patient says, "You get what I'm saying," then the patient's trusting you and you can show them anything. And they don't feel it as a threat—they don't feel it as an external explanation, it's not something external to be imposed on them, but something that, so that they kind of feel that there will be nothing opposed to them.

Although Dr. Ruiz emphasized the need for the clinician to approach the patient with openness as a means to facilitate trust, another psychiatrist, Dr. Ames, described the therapeutic relationship in more explicitly reciprocal terms:

I think things that help a therapeutic relationship work are when each is invested in the process. I feel like there are things I need to do and things the patient needs to do and for me I need to be open, curious, keep my ears open and not predetermine what's going to come out of my patient's mouth and be accepting of what he or she is saying. So for me to be active and engaged and interested in them and aware of my own feelings about either them or the content that they bring and how that colors my listening. And if I'm able to do that then I think we've got a good shot. Also I need to be consistent, I need to be professional, I need to be respectful and you know, be able to feel some sense of worth towards the patient. I think it's very hard if—it hasn't happened that many times—but if I really, really, really don't like somebody, it makes it hard. And I think in most patients I can find something to like and try to remember that they're in pain and coming for a particular reason. And then from the patient's perspective I think the things that I described earlier about what makes a good patient, in particular somebody who's interested, open, wants to learn about themselves, motivated, wants to feel better. Somewhere along that spectrum, even if they're not the ideal, you know, patient.

Dr. Ruiz also spoke of "motivated" patients—those who "know they need treatment and they want it"—as part of what makes a good clinical relationship.

In addition to a mutual engagement in the therapeutic process, other structural parameters appeared integral to positive clinical relationships. Of note, the patients and clinicians considered in this chapter were all part of (or anticipated) long-term treatment. Cathy, Mary, and Albert had each been seeing their current mental health providers for six to ten years; Rick expected to remain in therapy for at least a year. In fact, although Rick's insurance would only provide coverage for six months, he noted his willingness to pay out-of-pocket for continuing treatment, considering it worth "every penny." In addition to continuity, flexibility and availability were key characteristics of the manner in which these clinicians practiced. Dr. Ruiz was directly accessible by phone to his patients and told of one patient who finds solace "just knowing that she could get hold of somebody." Dr. Ames accommodated the work schedule of one of her patients by arranging to see him earlier than her usual hours.

Recognition in Clinical Relationships

Having presented a selection of narrative accounts, in the remainder of this chapter I turn to a preliminary framework for theorizing clinical relationships that are subjectively experienced as positive. Judith Butler's (2005) formulation of the self and her discussion of recognition in *Giving an Account of Oneself* may be useful as a conceptual model for thinking about positive clinical relationships. In this text, Butler writes against a certain formulation of the self as individualistic as well as transparent and, thus, knowable. Butler draws on a philosophical tradition that includes Levinas and Arendt refracted through feminist philosopher Adriana Cavarero to posit the fundamental relationality and opacity of the self. To bring her ideas closer to home, Butler's formation of self echoes Edward Sapir's theorization of the individual in relation to the world, defining the individual as "that total world of form, meaning, and implication of symbolic behavior which a given individual partly knows and directs, partly intuits and yields to, partly is ignorant of and is swayed by" (1949, 156). For Sapir, as for Butler, the self is forged in the interactive space between individuals.

Such a view of the self as constituted through relationships and as opaque, Butler argues, holds "a specific implication for an ethical bearing toward the other" (2005, 20). It is in this interactive space that Butler theorizes the dynamics of recognition. Drawing on Adriana Cavarero, Butler writes, "The question most central to recognition is a direct one, and it is addressed to the other: 'Who are you?' This question assumes that there is an other before us whom we do not know and cannot fully apprehend" (2005, 31).

This resounding question—who are you?—is a crucial one for therapeutics and, particularly, I think, for mental health care because the self is fully implicated in mental, behavioral, and emotional problems (compare Estroff et al. 1991). The question—who are you?—appears to be at the heart of the experiences of the patients and clinicians I have presented in this chapter. This is the question continually being asked, albeit implicitly, in the context of the clinical relationship. The dynamics and conditions of recognition consist in the time taken in the encounter, in remembering details of context, in continuity, in listening and bearing silences, and in the ineffable—what one feels "chest to chest, breast to breast." In the context of a continuous, long-term clinical relationship, it appears that even the seemingly perfunctory tasks of monitoring a patient's symptoms and daily functioning may be, as Cathy attests, experienced as "good doc-toring." The dynamics of recognition may also transcend the dyadic rela-tion, extending to the institutional level, as Albert described the clinic as "my home."

The question—who are you?—is not asked in order to classify. It is not a question of diagnosis or one of symptoms. By placing this question at the center of practice, these clinicians elide what Foucault describes in *The Birth of the Clinic* as the fundamental shift from a concern with "How do you feel?" to a concern with "Where does it hurt?" that marks modern medicine (1973). Positive clinical relationships seem not to have been eclipsed by the trend identified by Foucault. By positing that the self and, by extension, the other cannot be fully known, a logic of care based on recognition runs counter to the spectral gaze of biomedicine. Uncertainty and opacity are repositioned as fundamental conditions of, rather than impediments to, the therapeutic process. Adopting such a stance, clini-cians need to remain, as Dr. Ames articulates, "open, curious . . . and not predetermine what's going to come out of my patient's mouth." For patients, a level of uncertainty is, perhaps surprisingly, welcome. Albert's preference "for a doctor who doesn't know everything" resonates with Butler's assertion that recognition may "constitute a disposition of humil-ity and generosity alike" (2005, 42).

By continuing to ask "Who are you?" the clinician is introduced to greater and greater specificity and singularity, a point echoed by Paul Verhaeghe, who masterfully articulates the fundamental differences between medical and clinical psychodiagnostics:

> Unlike what takes place in medical diagnostics, [in psychodiagnostics] one cannot similarly bind a number of isolated symptoms into an objec-tive, universalizable syndrome that holds for just about every case. To the contrary, the more information the diagnostician acquires, the more specific the situation becomes, to the effect that generalization becomes all the more difficult. In medical diagnostics the symptoms are inter-preted as *signs* pointing to an underlying disturbance that can be both isolated and generalized. In clinical psychodiagnostics we are confronted with *signifiers* that carry endlessly shifting meanings in any given inter-action between the patient and the Other. . . . The universal element is missing; the clinical psychodiagnostic process results in a category in which N=1. The clinical psychodiagnostic questions are thus not so much 'What disease does this patient have?' but 'To whom or what do the symptoms refer? What are their meanings and functions, and who do they relate to?' There must be an underlying and, as yet, invisible struc-ture determining the whole that intersects in the patient. (2004, 5–6)

In a similar vein, John Strauss writes that "life is in the details. Life is specific, not general. There is nothing general about life" (1994, 106) and Kleinman observes that "in the context of chronic disorder, the illness becomes embodied in a particular life trajectory, environed in a concrete life world" (1988, 31). Yet—and here is the paradox—the recognition is never complete, but instead exists on an ever-elusive horizon. Drawing on Cavarero, Butler writes that the ethical stance thus consists "in asking the question, 'Who are you?' and continuing to ask it without any expectation of a full or final answer. The other to whom I pose this question will not be captured by any answer that might arrive to satisfy it. So if there is, in the question, a desire for recognition, this desire will be under an obligation to keep itself alive as desire and not to resolve itself" (2005, 43).

The clinicians described in this chapter appear to suspend the positivist impulse embedded in contemporary medicine that seeks to tame uncertainty.

Recognition in Contexts of Diversity

The ethical stance outlined by Butler, to desire recognition "without any expectation of a full or final answer," may be important for all patients, and may point the way toward "a more informed universalism." But this imperative may be intensified in the contemporary context of health-care delivery in which clinicians are likely to treat patients who may have limited English-language proficiency, have different care-seeking behaviors, and hold different expectations for care (Betancourt et al. 2005). With increasing diversity among clinical populations, the question "Who are you?" comes to the fore more obviously as clinicians may be confronted with unfamiliar complaints or different orientations to care. The proliferation of cultural competence efforts in medical education and practice reflects a growing awareness of shifts in patient demographics as well as health disparities borne by minority and low-income populations. As a response to increasingly diverse patient populations, cultural competence efforts challenge "one-size-fits-all health care" (Brach and Fraserirector 2000).

It would appear, at first blush, that efforts to provide culturally competent care align with decades of anthropological and cultural psychiatric research calling for awareness of local conceptions of illness that may differ from Western biomedical approaches. However, serious critiques have been leveled at cultural competence efforts on the basis of unsophisticated understandings of culture. Anthropological critiques assert that cultural competence models tend to present culture as static, treat culture as a variable, conflate culture with race-ethnicity, do not acknowledge diversity within groups, may inadvertently place blame on a patient's culture, often emphasize cultural difference, thereby obscuring structural power imbalances, and finally fail to recognize biomedicine as a cultural system itself (Good et al. 2003; Carpenter-Song, Nordquest, and

Longhofer 2007; Good and Hannah 2010; Kleinman and Benson 2006; Santiago-Irizarry 1996; Shaw 2005; Taylor 2003).

These critiques bear directly on how the central question of recognition—who are you?—will be configured in clinical encounters with diverse populations. Reductive approaches to this question, exemplified by cultural competence efforts, approach difference through crude classifications that reify existing categories not to ask "who are you?" but to claim "I know who you are!"

In contrast, the approach I am advocating, drawing on the concept of recognition and grounded in the experiences of patients and clinicians, facilitates approaching difference and otherness through openness. Butler's formulation appears to hold specific relevance for the negotiation of difference in cross-cultural encounters, as she writes, "An ability to affirm what is contingent and incoherent in oneself may allow one to affirm others who may or may not 'mirror' one's own constitution" (2005, 41).

With such openness comes the opportunity for surprise, as Dr. Ames explains her confrontation with her own cultural biases:

> I became aware of my own preconceived notions about him. And being a young Caucasian man from a pretty—not wealthy but comfortable—family growing up in a wealthy area, gone to good schools, and I kind of had an idea of how he might respond to me being a black woman. And then when he disclosed that he had spent time in Kenya and that his family had actually welcomed a young man from Kenya who's living with the family, I found myself relaxing a bit and thinking, "Okay maybe we'll be okay." So I've had to be aware of my own cultural biases.

Rather than a skill to be learned or a set of facts to be committed to memory, recognition implies a stance, an inclination toward the other that desires to know but understands the utter impossibility of realizing that longing.

The Political Economy of Care

Although it focuses on the patient-clinician dyad and institutional cultures of care, the study is also positioned more broadly in relation to the current environment of health-care delivery in the United States. It is imperative to contextualize the dynamics of recognition considered in this chapter in order to interrogate structural constraints on, and threats to, the provision of what patients and clinicians consider to be good care. Although a full discussion is beyond the scope of this chapter, I wish to note briefly that dimensions of the political economy of care have percolated through our conversations with patients and clinicians. In a health-care climate increasingly favoring short-term and pharmaceutically based therapies, the experiences described by the patients and clinicians in this chapter appear to happen very much in spite of the contemporary trends in health-care delivery. The patients introduced in this chapter were all fortunate to have either adequate insurance, with coverage for mental health care, or government-subsidized care. Even so, clinicians spoke of "tweaking" official diagnoses to "get the patient what he needs," such as coverage for additional sessions. The clinicians in this chapter were acutely aware of a fragile balance to provide patients with the best care while abiding strict rules and regulations imposed by insurers, a point Dr. Ames articulated: "I mean the thing that's always on my mind in doing psychotherapy with patients is how long will the treatment be funded by the insurer and I think I talked about this with the other patient. And [that patient] has a biologically based diagnosis so I don't anticipate any problems but that is always, you know, in the back of our minds about how to have the treatment paid for."

Thus, although the relationships described in this chapter offer a model toward which to strive, it remains the case that much of what mediates experiences and outcomes of health care falls outside of the dyadic inter-actions of patients and clinicians. In a recent commentary, Jim Kim cri-tiqued what he describes as the "work around culture" of contemporary American medicine that depends on the abilities and willingness of "heroic doctors" to "work around" broken systems of health-care deliv-ery (2008). Heroism, I heartily agree, is not a solvent strategy for the long term. The dynamics of recognition are, at some level, a product of serendipity—whatever makes a connection click—but certainly seem less likely to occur outside of contexts that allow for continuity and flex-ibility. Patients and clinicians can only be as good as the conditions in which they practice. The high stakes of cultivating good clinical relation-ships demand that such relationships not be left wholly to chance or accident. Structural reforms would require rethinking bureaucratized managed care to foster the conditions of possibility for the emergence of a new logic of care based on recognition (for further consideration of health-care bureaucracy and health-care economics, see chapter 9, this volume).

Conclusion

Clinical relationships mediated by recognition disrupt the (usual) assump-tion of a fundamental split between patients and clinicians. Positively experienced clinical relationships are not a battle in which patients must struggle to have their voices heard and their experiences taken seriously. Rather than seeking to bound or contain the experiences of their patients, the clinicians described appear to maintain openness to uncertainty, plac-ing contingency and opacity at the heart of the clinical encounter. I am heartened by their experiences and encouraged that the "Walmart-ing of American psychiatry," as Alistair Donald (2001) describes it, is not totalizing even in mainstream mental health practices. Further study of positive clinical relationships is called for to push back against rationalized, reductionist care and to advocate for what may really work.

Notes

1. I do not have information on the class backgrounds of clinicians.
2. Interviews are conducted separately with patients and clinicians.

References

Betancourt, Joseph R., Alexander R. Green, J. Emilio Carrillo, and Elyse R. Park. 2005. "Cultural Competence and Health Care Disparities: Key Perspectives and Trends." *Health Affairs* 24(2): 499–505.

Brach, Cindy, and Irene Fraserirector. 2000. "Can Cultural Competency Reduce Racial and Ethnic Health Disparities? A Review and Conceptual Model." *Medical Care Research and Review* 57(4): 181–217.

Butler, Judith. 2005. *Giving an Account of Oneself.* New York: Fordham University Press.

Carpenter-Song, Elizabeth. 2009. "Caught in the Psychiatric Net: Meanings and Experiences of ADHD, Pediatric Bipolar Disorder, and Mental Health Treatment Among Families in the United States." *Culture, Medicine and Psychiatry* 33(1): 61–85.

Carpenter-Song, Elizabeth, Megan Nordquest, and Jeffrey Longhofer. 2007. "Cultural Competence Reexamined: Critique and Directions for the Future." *Psychiatric Services* 58(10): 1362–365.

Carpenter-Song, Elizabeth, Edward Chu, Robert Drake, Mieka Ritsema, Beverly Smith, and Hoyt Alverson. 2010. "Ethno-Cultural Variations in the Experience and Meaning of Mental Illness and Treatment: Implications for Access and Utilization." *Transcultural Psychiatry* 47(2): 224–51.

Cicourel, Aaron. 1983. "Hearing Is Not Believing: Language and the Structure of Belief in Medical Communication." In *The Social Organization of Doctor-Patient Communication,* edited by Alexander Dundas Todd and Sue Fisher. Washington, D.C.: Center for Applied Linguistics.

Coyle, Joanne. 1999. "Exploring the Meaning of 'Dissatisfaction' with Health Care: The Importance of 'Personal Identity Threat.' " *Sociology of Health and Illness* 21(1): 95–123.

Donald, Alistair. 2001. "The Wal-marting of American Psychiatry: An Ethnography of Psychiatric Practice in the Late 20th Century." *Culture Medicine and Psychiatry* 25(4): 427–39.

Estroff, Sue, William S. Lachicotte, Linda C. Illingworth, and Anna Johnston. 1991. "Everybody's Got a Little Mental Illness: Accounts of Illness and Self among People with Severe, Persistent Mental Illnesses." *Medical Anthropology Quarterly* 5(4): 331–69.

Fisher, Sue, and Stephen Groce. 1990. "Accounting Practices in Medical Interviews." *Language in Society* 19(2): 225–50.

Foucault, Michel. 1973. *The Birth of the Clinic: An Archaeology of Medical Perception.* New York: Vintage Books.

Good, Byron J. 1994. *Medicine, Rationality, and Experience.* New York: Cambridge University Press.

Good, Mary-Jo DelVecchio. 1995. *American Medicine: The Quest for Competence.* Berkeley: University of California Press.

Good, Mary-Jo DelVecchio, and Seth Hannah. 2010. "Medical Cultures." In *Handbook of Cultural Sociology,* edited by John R. Hall, Laura Grindstaff, and Ming-Cheng M. Lo. London: Routledge.

Good, Mary-Jo DelVecchio, Byron J. Good, Cynthia Schaffer, and Stuart E. Lind. 1990. "American Oncology and the Discourse on Hope." *Culture, Medicine and Psychiatry* 14(1): 59–79.

Good, Mary-Jo DelVecchio, Cara James, Byron J. Good, and Adrienne E. Becker. 2003. "The Culture of Medicine and Racial, Ethnic, and Class Disparities in Healthcare." In *Unequal Treatment: Confronting Racial and Ethnic Disparities in Health Care,* edited by Brian D. Smedley, Adrienne Y. Stith, and Alan Ray Nelson. Washington, D.C.: National Academies Press.

Jenkins, Janis H., and Elizabeth A. Carpenter-Song. 2005. "The New Paradigm of Recovery from Schizophrenia: Cultural Conundrums of Improvement Without Cure." *Culture, Medicine and Psychiatry* 29(4): 379–413.

Kim, Jim Yong. 2008. "Commentary on Keynote Address by Arthur Kleinman, 'Culture and Caregiving: How I See Medical Anthropology and Global Mental Health.'" Critical Research on Culture, Psychiatry, and Mental Health Services: Celebrating a Quarter Century of the Harvard NIMH Medical Anthropology Training Program. Harvard Medical School, Cambridge, Mass. (May 16–17).

Kleinman, Arthur. 1988. *The Illness Narratives: Suffering, Healing, and the Human Condition.* New York: Basic Books.

Kleinman, Arthur, and Peter Benson. 2006. "Anthropology in the Clinic: The Problem of Cultural Competency and How to Fix It." *PLoS Medicine* 3(10): 1673–676.

Mishler, Elliot. 1984. *The Discourse of Medicine: The Dialectics of Medical Interviews.* Norwood, N.J.: Ablex.

Santiago-Irizarry, Vilma. 1996. "Culture as Cure." *Cultural Anthropology* 11(1): 3–24.

Sapir, Edward. 1949. *Culture, Language and Personality: Selected Essays.* Berkeley: University of California Press.

Shaw, Susan J. 2005. "The Politics of Recognition in Culturally Appropriate Care." *Medical Anthropology Quarterly* 19(3): 290–309.

Smedley, Brian E., Adrienne Y. Stith, and Alan Ray Nelson. 2003. *Unequal Treatment: Confronting Ethnic and Racial Disparities in Health Care.* Washington, D.C.: National Academies Press.

Strauss, John S. 1994. "The Person with Schizophrenia as Person II: Approaches to the Subjective and Complex." *British Journal of Psychiatry* 164(supp. 23): 103–07.

Taylor, Janelle. S. 2003. "The Story Catches You and You Fall Down: Tragedy, Ethnography, and 'Cultural Competence.'" *Medical Anthropology Quarterly* 17(2): 159–81.

U.S. Department of Health and Human Services (HHS). 2001. *Mental Health: Culture, Race, Ethnicity—Supplement to Mental Health: Report of the Surgeon General*. Rockville, Md.: Government Printing Office.

Verhaeghe, Paul. 2004. *On Being Normal and Other Disorders: A Manual for Clinical Psychodiagnostics*. New York: Other Press.

West, Candace. 1984a. "When the Doctor is a 'Lady': Power, Status and Gender in Physician-Patient Encounters." *Symbolic Interaction* 7(1): 87–105.

———. 1984b. *Routine Complications: Troubles with Talk Between Doctors and Patients*. Bloomington: Indiana University Press.

West, Candace, and Richard Frankel. 1991. "Miscommunication in Medicine." In *Miscommunication and Problematic Talk*, edited by Nikolas Coupland, Howard Giles, and John M. Wiemann. Newbury Park, Calif.: Sage Publications.

Young, Katherine. 1997. *Presence in the Flesh: The Body in Medicine*. Cambridge, Mass.: Harvard University Press.

Chapter 9

"The Culture of Medicine" As Revealed in Patients' Perspectives on Psychiatric Treatment

T HE INTRODUCTION to this volume notes a shift in emphasis from the patient's cultural background to the culture of medicine in explanations of the production of disparities in care (Good et al. 2003). This shift reflects the development of a more complex and encompassing understanding of culture, one that goes beyond the equation of culture with the pentad of racial-ethnic categories of identity and encompasses the cultural orientations and assumptions of medical institutions. Given this new focus, the questions we asked patients in the study included a contextual explanation: "We are trying to understand the experience of treating patients with various cultural backgrounds and practices, but we are also very interested in the culture of clinical practice itself."

Mental health treatment in the United States has become increasingly standardized, rationalized, manualized (encoded in the instructions of a how-to manual), and regulated, with bureaucratic and economic considerations often eclipsing the goal of delivering quality healthcare (Hopper 2001; Kirschner and Lachicotte 2001; Calabrese 2008; Silverman 1996). With the growth of psychopharmacology and other biologically reductionist frameworks of treatment, the voices of patients have been marginalized in many areas of mental health treatment. For example, psychiatrists typically meet with patients only long enough to check medication effects and side effects. The psychiatric clinician is frequently immersed in diagnostic checklists, lab tests, and insurance reimbursement forms rather than in narratives of patient experiences.

In light of the theoretical literature, the situation is both Foucauldian and Weberian. It is the product of radical changes in medical practice involving the development of a "medical gaze" that separates the patient's body from his or her personal identity (Foucault 1973) and treats the objectified body within a standardized and routinized, and frequently impersonal, bureaucratic organizational structure (Weber 1946). The situation is also economic, reflecting the influence of capitated managed care systems and other innovations in health-care funding.

In this context, anthropological studies can allow patients' voices to be heard, informing clinicians and policymakers as well as providing insights into the local effects of more global changes in healthcare economics and modes of practice. Our study focused on several institutions in the Boston area that are exemplary in the attention they pay to the patient's perspective. As Elizabeth Carpenter-Song points out in chapter 8 of this volume, many of the patients interviewed for this study describe their relationships with their current health-care providers in very positive terms. However, it is still useful to look at the more negative stories told by patients in an effort to understand the effects of the Foucauldian and Weberian forces at work and to identify potential barriers to treatment.

The goal of this chapter is to immerse the reader in patient narratives of their psychiatric treatment in order to understand their perspectives on the culture of medicine, especially what they identify as good care and bad care. Primary attention will be focused on negative experiences and other factors that may serve as barriers to health care and that can guide our improvements of the health-care system.

During my involvement in this anthropological research into clinical contexts, I felt simultaneously a cultural insider and an outsider. In addition to my anthropological training, I have training in clinical psychology and several years of experience in health care, including a clinical fellowship at one of Harvard's teaching hospitals. My internship at the Chicago-Read Mental Health Center, a large state mental hospital, immersed me in many patients' unfavorable views of their treatment, many reasonable—especially in cases of coerced treatment—and some reflecting psychotic distortions.

I chose to undertake simultaneous training in anthropology and clinical psychology primarily to understand human lives in a holistic, nonreductive way. This training, however, was also aimed at a better understanding of disciplinary differences and conflicts. I have often spoken of my anthropologist side and my clinician side in discussions with my students at University College London and the University of Chicago, especially when one of these voices asserts itself in a particular exchange. In examining the patient narratives for this chapter, I found, within my interdisciplinary approach, a tension between the relativistic view of anthropology, which tends to privilege the insider's view of any particular group, and the diagnostic view of the clinical sciences, in which "what a patient says may be considered a symptom of mental illness instead of an opinion to be incorporated into health care planning" (Velpry 2008, 241). This chapter intentionally limits itself to a description of the insider's view to avoid indulging in armchair diagnosis of patients who are not under my care.

There were also inner conflicts within my clinician side. I have been trained in the empathic exploration of intensely personal experiences and emotions with people who are destabilized and vulnerable. I have also been trained in noninjurious methods of taking down and restraining a violent patient within the context of (frequently coerced) inpatient treatment. Psychiatric treatment is thus a combination of compassion and coercion. Coercive interventions have produced many critics who argue that psychiatric treatment is simply the punishment of social deviance. However, I have also known very compassionate and ethical clinicians, very ill and self-destructive patients, and many appreciative patients, some of whom began their relationship with me or another clinician in such a dark place that they evaluated everything around them negatively, including the prospect of a continuing existence.

Given these disciplinary tensions and inner conflicts, it was sometimes difficult to document the negative characterizations of health care given by some patients. The clinician side of my personality felt uneasy and I was concerned that hard-working and well-intentioned doctors with expanding caseloads would feel unjustly attacked. However, this chapter is motivated by a genuine interest and concern, deriving from my own clinical practice, in how patients view their treatment and a belief that negative experiences are important for clinicians to understand as potential barriers to future treatment. Even in those cases in which the patient making the negative statement is experiencing a psychotic episode or is otherwise confused about things, the rough edges of psychiatric treatment may be revealed in a useful way that allows clinicians to improve health-care services.

The patients we interviewed for this study discussed positive and negative experiences with doctors at the clinical facilities involved in the study. They also discussed experiences at other clinical facilities not involved in this study and sometimes spoke hypothetically about good or bad care. I coded all these characterizations of providers in the interview transcripts to assemble a list of qualities that patients associate with negative clinical experiences and positive clinical experiences. I refer to individual patients using pseudonyms.

How Do Patients Define Positive Treatment Experiences?

The most frequently mentioned characteristic of a good therapeutic relationship was the clinician's ability to communicate effectively. This included not only being able to listen but also being able to give opinions and advice useful to the patient. Edward described his therapist as "interactive but sympathetic" and felt that he was lucky to have found such a person. Ann, when asked how she would define a good doctor, said, "It would be someone that you're able to listen to and also that they ask you questions and take the things so it's like a two-way conversation . . . to listen and also have a conversation . . . those are the doctors I think are good." When asked the same question, another patient, Alice, said, "It would be one that the doctor spends enough time to hear what you have to say and you listen to him also for his advice and you are able to tell him, you know, some of the things that you don't like doing and he may not agree with it but he respects your opinion about it."

Patrick mentioned that a clinician with whom he has recently started working has done a really good job of listening to him and understanding his situation, but that he would now like to hear more of her opinion: "I was kind of edging towards, recently, towards having her give me more of her perspective . . . so that's what I'm looking for from her, going forward. And she responded to that with an answer that I was satisfied with."

Other patients gave positive descriptions of clinicians who provided useful advice on relationships, helped the patient look at a situation objectively and figure out why she was confused, repeated certain things the patient said in a way that gave him more awareness, knew how to ask the right questions, and encouraged patients to discuss if they had any problems with the therapy. Many characterized a good clinician as someone who makes you feel comfortable in discussing very personal issues. As Edward said, "I go to tell her things that I can't tell anyone else which is wonderful. I can say exactly what I'm feeling . . . and the feelings that I'm not proud of."

This type of trusting relationship was easier to establish if the patient felt that the clinician was caring, kind, genuinely concerned about the patient, and ethical. Several patients described good clinicians as being dedicated to the patient, keeping up with what's happening in the patient's life, spending enough time during sessions rather than rushing, and returning phone calls.

Another prominent theme was the view that a good clinician treats you like a person, with the word *person* sometimes contrasted with the word *patient*. When Julie was asked what she liked about her doctor, she replied, "She looks at me as a person." In contrast, Ruth reported that staff at her hospital made her feel "like I'm less than a person" and Nora that certain psychiatrists with whom she had worked in the past viewed her "as a patient-like person."

The narratives reviewed here provide useful indications of what patients understand to be competent clinical care. Patients in this study described good therapeutic relationships as those characterized by an interactive communication that blends listening and active problem-solving and by the patient being treated "as a person." This characterization of a good clinician as treating you like a person implies a critique of a particular sort of clinical care: a dehumanizing descent into the role of the patient lost in an impersonal health-care bureaucracy. In the following sections, we focus on negative characterizations of clinical encounters revealed in interviews with patients.

Negative Experiences with the Health-Care System and Doctors

The patient contemplating mental health services faces many potential difficulties that make the process daunting and may lead the patient to avoid health-care services completely. In the interviews completed for this project, several patients described negative experiences with the health-care system and doctors as a barrier to seeking subsequent care. Patients also discussed the distrust they feel for an increasingly impersonal medical system geared toward the technological treatment of physical disease rather than the more interpersonally oriented healing of illness (Eisenberg 1977). This distrust includes suspicions about the economic and government connections of the health-care system, and doctors are sometimes described as uncaring and motivated by their own economic interests. Other narratives discuss psychiatric illness stigma, the destabilizing effects of discrimination, inequality in treatment options, and poor institutional responses to cultural diversity.

The most prominent aspects of negative clinical encounters patients discussed depicted clinicians with inflated egos viewing patients as specimens or subjects rather than human beings and being either authoritarian or formulaic (such as quickly and automatically prescribing medications) without any obvious concern for the patient. Several patients mentioned that an encounter with such a clinician gave them a negative impression of the entire hospital or caused them to avoid seeking treatment generally.

Stan, a patient at a large teaching hospital, said, "When the team comes into your room, there are some who treat you like a specimen, not a good thing." Julie describes a similar feeling at her former hospital:

> I felt like a subject, like cattle. I was seeing a neurologist there, and he was slumped over the computer and asked me, "So, have I ever seen you before?" And I said, "Yeah, three months ago." "So what's the problem?"

"Well, I'm walking a little funny." He told me to walk. So I walked for him, and he said, "You seem to be the same to me!" This guy didn't even remember me, and then he had the nerve to fake that he knew how I walked. . . . They're kind of on this big ego trip.

More than one patient had the feeling that their clinician was just going through the motions to collect a paycheck:

[They're] just writing you off and just doing what they have to do and not looking further to see if they can help you become whole and function the way you should function or could. Or are they just treating you because you're there and you have an appointment and you have Medicare and you have insurance, whatever? You have to wonder sometimes. (Alice)

I felt like he was more interested in collecting a paycheck than in care. And I know that doesn't sound good, but that's how I felt. It was, "Here, come in" and "Let's get your 'scrips" and "You can go." . . . He just wasn't interested in anything other than writing the prescriptions. (Angela)

These statements resonate with Gray's discussion of the managed care era's transformation of the doctor-patient relationship from a personal relationship into "a quasi-business transaction" (Gray 1997, 34). As Angela's statement indicates, many patients interpret an exclusive focus on medication, without the development of a therapeutic conversation, to be a form of clinical neglect:

It was just a medication thing. They just kept adding medications. . . . I never had a psychiatrist here that I could tell things to. Like all the other ones were like [pause] . . . how to explain it? . . . They saw you as a patient-like person. I guess that's what it is. (Nora)

I think that's all he knows is medications! I don't think he's a well-rounded person at all. . . . I don't see no difference between these drugs and the drugs on the street! (Irene)

In contrast to positive characterizations, specifically those that describe a situation of effective bidirectional communication in which the clinician listens but also shares advice and guidance, two patients complained that their therapists just listened and didn't actively seek out the relevant issues or provide guidance:

I thought he didn't really get to what my issues were. . . . He listened most of the time. Basically just listened. [Laughs.] Talked a little bit but not much. So that's what I've had previously. (Edward)

I would joke with myself and with a few other people that . . . this doctor or therapist had a pretty good deal. Because I'd show up for forty-five minutes to fifty minutes, once a week, and she'd hear me tell some good stories. 'Cause I'd try to, because it was my first time going to therapy, I didn't exactly feel comfortable disclosing some of the darker things that I'd been dealing with. So at times I'd try to make things more light. So I feel like basically it was like story-time for fifty minutes. And she got paid handsomely for me doing that. She employed the method of just long, still pauses, just letting me talk. And I can put myself in a room for fifty minutes and talk if I want to. But I think I was looking more for some perspective and guidance. . . . And maybe I should have been more forthright in asking for that. And I just, I guess it's, she embodied many of the stereotypes that get poked fun at, as far as what therapists are. Stuff you see in the movies. Or TV, that kind of thing. I couldn't help, at the time, thinking it was a little bit ironic, funny. But at the same time, disappointing that I couldn't, I wasn't finding what I wanted to find. (Patrick)

An important phenomenon revealed in the interviews is a situation in which a single negative experience is transferred to an entire institution or to the process of seeking psychiatric services generally. In this way, negative clinical experiences can be a barrier to seeking care in the future. Julie, who described the incident in which a clinician who could not remember meeting her stated that her walking had not changed, admits that her negative feelings about her previous hospital are based on this particular doctor, "which probably isn't fair." Another patient, Ann, transferred her experience at one small hospital to the category of all small hospitals: "I have no trust in doctors in small hospitals right now. . . . I feel like, you're a guinea pig. . . . I just have probably had a bad experience and am very bitter with them." Describing a negative experience with a clinician in Puerto Rico, Pablo stated,

This first doctor, I don't know, maybe he didn't mean it, maybe he was not aware, but I felt like he was kind of a little bit rude with me, so I didn't like that, so I felt like, wow, if this is the person that I'm going to talk about my emotional problems, so I'd rather deal with my problems on my own . . . I saw him once and I didn't go ever again. . . . I didn't want to seek treatment.

Patrick says that his previous therapist had her own private office ("I guess it was . . . more what I expected to encounter when I went to therapy. Nicely decorated office, leather couch, bunch of academic books on the shelf"). However, he explains that he actually feels more comfortable at his hospital because of his relationship with his doctor:

It has everything to do with my relationship with Dr. Jackson. She could be somewhere else—in the first environment that I was in the first time that I went to therapy—and if I had that same connection with my therapist, I'd probably see that whole environment in a different way too. (Patrick)

This section has described patients' interpretations of clinical encounters in which a collaborative relationship marked by trust and effective bidirectional communication was not reached. Instead, clinical care was interpreted as an impersonal business transaction in which the dispensing of medications substituted for a supportive relationship in which useful advice is shared. The Foucauldian themes of objectification and depersonalization are prominent. In the descriptions of doctors who are exclusively concerned with medicating the underlying biological disease and ignoring the person, one is reminded of the anthropologist Susan DiGiacomo's description of her own feeling of being an ignored bystander as the medical system conducted its war directly against the disease entity within her (1987). DiGiacomo, who was diagnosed with Hodgkin's lymphoma during her dissertation research, writes that clinicians found her desire to understand her illness and its treatment inappropriate. One doctor commented that he did not think it was wise for DiGiacomo to try to become an expert on her own disease because it could be psychologically damaging. Rather than being engaged as a participant in her own treatment, DiGiacomo felt reduced to a biological organism, the battlefield on which doctors waged their "war on cancer." She was depersonalized. Robert Desjarlais (2000) has also described this diminished sense of personhood among people with mental illness (often a result of how others stigmatize and ignore them) as well as the ability of supportive contexts to help restore this sense of personhood.

Distrust of the Health-Care System and Its Economic and Government Connections

In addition to distrust of particular clinicians and, by association, their particular hospitals, several patients also expressed distrust in the health-care system as a whole given its economic and government connections:

> There's a couple theories. One, they have a deal with the people that make the drugs . . . we'll supply you all these drugs that you want at a very cheap price, but these are the drugs you prescribe to your patients. Insurance is another theory. . . . we won't cover that drug, so you can't give it to our patients. (Ted)

Another patient, Julie, expressed an extreme distrust of insurance companies and fear that information about her sexuality in hospital records could be used against her by the government:

> Julie: I don't like insurance companies. Because of privacy. I don't like the thing that's going on in our country with reality shows. They're preparing us! . . . With these insurance companies, suddenly you're a medical record. You have this disease. It's like putting yourself in a box. . . . I'm gay, but I don't tell the insurance company about my sexuality.

Q: But you're comfortable telling your social worker?

Julie: Yeah.

Q: You just ask that she doesn't write it in the chart.

Julie: Right.

Q: Why is that?

Julie: Well, like if we get another Republican in office they're going to come and exterminate all the gay people. [Laughs, a little uneasily]

The economics behind unequal treatment of the rich and the poor was a concern for Alice, who stated that every time she goes to the emergency room at her hospital, she never sees people who look well off, only poor people. She wonders about the rich people—"Where do they go? ... I never see them in this institution"—and is told by her family, "Well, maybe they have an in-road." Having once waited ten hours for care in an emergency room, Alice complained: "Do the doctors just have a special deal with them? What is going on?"

Reflecting on their studies of doctor-patient relationships, Mary-Jo Good and Byron Good (2000) argue that contemporary studies of doctor-patient communications should focus on how these relationships mediate larger relations of culture, knowledge, and power, including globalized political economies of medicine. It seems clear that many of the problems identified in the previous section may be related not only to the development of new psychopharmacological and diagnostic technologies but also to the restructuring of American medical care around capitated managed care systems. Interposed between the doctor and patient are new, ethically questionable physician incentive systems, impersonal rules that result in denials of care, and even gag orders through which managed care systems limit the information that doctors can give their patients relevant to their treatment. All these innovations have undermined patient trust in doctors and have caused many patients to conclude that doctors are agents of the state or the managed care company rather than the ally of patients (Mechanic 1997; Gray 1997).

Stigma Within and Beyond Clinical Services

In his report on mental health (U.S. Department of HHS 1999, 3), the Surgeon General identified stigma as "the most formidable obstacle to future progress in the arena of mental illness and health." People who could potentially benefit from psychiatric services are often put off by the fact that seeking these services may result in social stigma. Nora mentioned that she hates to tell people that she suffers from depression.

She explains, "It's kind of like it's taboo." However, she also says that a summer spent hospitalized helped her to realize to what extent she had also internalized these stigmatizing understandings of mental illness:

> Well, you know . . . as soon as I walked in, it was like, there was all these really creepy looking people, just like, "Oh, man!" Like, "I really don't belong here." But then, once you get to meet people and talk to people, it's like everybody's got a background. Like everybody, regardless of how they look, they still have a story to tell. And I think, if anything, I learned it's not to pass judgment on people. Based on what they look like. And it bothers me if I'm with somebody and they do it.

When asked if her co-workers knew that she was seeking therapy, Ann explained:

> Ann: I keep that to myself. You know, even my husband's sisters don't know. I've just kept that between the three of us. . . . I don't think people really understand that much about it. . . . They don't look at it like an illness. It's getting a bad rep.
>
> Q: As opposed to an illness what do people think of it as?
>
> Ann: I don't know, something freaky or something, you know what I mean. It's not really accepted.

In my interview with Ashley, a Chinese American born in Shanghai, she said that an important aspect of her outpatient mental health treatment is that her parents do not know about it. Her parents would not understand, she explained, and many of her Asian friends strongly objected to her treatment because in many Asian cultures mental illness carries a stigma. She makes sure that her doctor sends her bill to her apartment rather than her parents' home:

> Ashley: It's kind of quack for them. So, quack doctors. Also, the stigma of having some kind of mental illness. I mean, I function fine in society most times. So, for them it's better to hide it than to seek help and for them the help is sort of non-legitimized. You know, it's not a doctor who does operations. It's a different thing. So, they still don't know about it. I have one very close friend who fought me for it. I have some friends who are very supportive of it.
>
> Q: Is that a pretty typical pattern within people from Shanghai?
>
> Ashley: Oh, yeah! And in Asian culture overall. It's sort of taboo. We don't talk about it. Like, unless you go completely bonkers and he knows something is wrong and then you get committed, basically. Then you have shamed the family that we don't want to talk about it and just send you away somewhere.

Q: So, what would be their approach to handling some of the problems that you mentioned, such as depression or crying a lot?

Ashley: Soldier through it. Repress it.

These and other experiences of psychiatric stigma described in the study portray stigma as a pervasive aspect of patients' interpersonal contexts that threatens what is at stake for them and that is managed creatively using various strategies. This view of stigma, which emphasizes its interpersonal and cultural nature as well as the agency of stigmatized individuals, is in line with current anthropological understandings (Yang et al. 2007; Jenkins and Carpenter-Song 2008, 2009).

Importantly, psychiatric stigma was also found to be a factor within the context of clinical services. Emily states that clinicians at her hospital made medical errors due to prejudice. They made the assumption that, because she had a mental health treatment history, her complaints of abdominal pain were manifestations of a delusion:

It wasn't prejudice because of my race or my gender . . . it was prejudice because I'm mentally ill. [Laughs] And I had medical problems, and they just assumed that I was just crazy . . . gall-bladder that almost burst, and they put me in the inpatient psych for about five days, and in agony, and charted me down every time I complained and doubled over, that I was basically delusional. [Laughs] Great fun. And the surgeon said I almost died. [Laughs] I don't know why I laugh but it's over and I feel safe now so that's what makes it funny. (Emily)

This finding is in line with studies that reveal stigma in the interpretations of many health professionals as well as in the society more broadly (see, for example, Rao et al. 2009; Keane 1990). Emily's experience clearly shows the danger of equating a particular person with a particular diagnosis in a clinical setting.

Cultural and Gender Diversity and Similarity

The last potential barrier I discuss to seeking health-care services is the existence of cultural and gender differences between the patient and clinical staff. In this study, many patients who had a doctor from a cultural background or gender different from their own said it made no difference. Patrick, who sees a female African American clinician, felt that he was similar to her in his patience and that the ethnic and gender differences did not matter. Edward said that he was not even sure whether his clinician was "white or African American or some combination" and that it makes no difference to him:

I just don't really think about that difference, I guess. . . . I mean, there's nothing that would make me not want to say something. . . . I've had to talk about you know, sensitive things like sexual stuff, you know both from disease and history and stuff. There's been no problem there.

Another example demonstrates that, for a particular Asian patient, having a non-Asian clinician was not a problem. In fact, Ashley feels that having an Asian clinician, specifically a male Asian clinician, would have been a problem.

> Ashley: I think it's probably more useful to talk to someone who is not from my background. . . . I think that it might be difficult for someone like my mother to come and talk to someone who is, you know, Caucasian, basically. For me, I grew up with all my friends from different ethnicities. So, for me it's not really a big deal. There's no language barrier, I can express myself freely and I'm not inhibited by the fact that he's not Asian. . . . at one point Dr. D. asked me if I had any issue with him as a male figure because I have authority issues with males. I said, frankly, "No, because you're white."
>
> Q: So, it's limited to—
>
> Ashley: To Asian male figures.

Thus for Ashley, working with a therapist of a different gender was not a problem as long as the therapist was also from a different cultural background. Gender seemed to be a more important factor for Edward, and he preferred not to work with another male: "It's really not as easy for me to talk to men. There's always that kind of . . . opposition or aggression."

Two patients did have issues with cultural diversity: a Jewish woman and a Catholic nun. These issues, though, had to do with understanding of their religious practice. Ruth, a Jewish patient, who abstained from pork for religious reasons, experienced an inability of staff to provide her with an adequate meal:

> Well, because I'm Jewish, we had a big issue and it took them over a week and a half for them to not serve me pork. It was a big issue. . . . You'd think I was asking for the world on a platter. I just tried every single meal. What would happen, they would have chicken and they would have pork. But by the time I got through the line, I'd be stuck with the pork and no food. . . . And I also have a seafood allergy, and what would happen is, the alternative would be gone, and I would have to have the seafood. And all they were offering me were turkey and Swiss sandwiches, and after a week of eating turkey and Swiss sandwiches for lunch and dinner, you might get a little frustrated. You know what I'm saying?

Mary, a Catholic nun who is seeing a clinician at a large teaching hospital, also experienced a certain level of cultural misunderstanding:

> It's always hard for them especially if they're not Catholic or practicing Catholics to figure out what a nun is and all of the words like *superior* and *provincial* and the whole language barrier has to be over time transferred to the next person, so they can understand what you're talking about. . . . And I guess it's hard to, because they're not nuns, obviously they don't necessarily understand, they're trying really hard to understand your values. Like Katie . . . I said something and she said, "Oh, well, normally you would just go out and have safe sex with somebody," and I'm like it's not really an option. [Laughs] . . . Then I explained to her the whole story because she really, I don't think she had any clue as to what a religious sister was. So I, there's a lot of education that has to get done.

The data described in this section were useful in breaking the notion of cultural difference from a simplistic association with racial-ethnic identity. The patient experiences reviewed demonstrate that cultural difference can be a relevant barrier for particular white patients (those within minority religious traditions) and that having a clinician who does not match one's ethnicity can be irrelevant to patient satisfaction or even uniquely advantageous for certain nonwhite patients like Ashley. I am reminded of a patient I treated while working at the University of Chicago Hospitals. His family was from Calabria and his reaction to my last name—invoking his relationship with his father and other associations—almost prevented us from working together. In the end, we were able to work together in spite of his initial reaction. In this case, as in Ashley's, cultural similarity was the problem, which opens useful therapeutic possibilities for working through the problem but which can still be a very real barrier to clinical services.

Discussion

This chapter has explored the culture of medicine through analysis of the ways in which psychiatric patients describe positive and negative clinical encounters. The patients interviewed for this study tended to describe positive therapeutic interactions and relationships as those in which communication is easy, the clinician listens well but also offers opinions or advice, and seems available and genuinely concerned about the patient as a person. Negative therapeutic encounters included those in which the patient felt dehumanized, treated "like a specimen" or equated with a diagnostic category, given medication without communication, and treated by clinicians who are just going through the motions to collect a paycheck. These narratives resonate with a Foucauldian-Weberian critique of the culture of medicine in the United States.

These findings have many implications for improving clinical services and rebuilding trust between clinicians and patients. Health-care services can decrease the patient's feeling of being dehumanized in an impersonal health-care bureaucracy if they demonstrate a respect for the patient's human dignity and personal complexity, offer patients more opportunities for bidirectional communication with clinicians, and are aware of psychiatric stigma among patients and their families as well as in the attitudes and assumptions of clinical staff. These findings foreground the continuing importance of human relationships, personhood, meanings, communication, and trust to patients.

However, as Good and Good argue, issues such as trust in the context of clinician-patient relationships "cannot be adequately understood using models of a former era of research that focused narrowly on conversational aspects of doctor-patient communications" (2000, 255). New forces (capitated managed care systems) have positioned themselves between the doctor and patient, bringing impersonal rules from above that limit access to care and even limit the health-care-relevant information that doctors can share with their patients (Mechanic 1997). Thus even the content of doctor-patient communications becomes subject to bureaucratic control, exacerbating the growing distrust among patients that their doctors are agents of the state or the managed care company rather than the patient's ally.

The negative impact of these global structures on the dynamics of the doctor-patient relationship has been a concern for many scholars, and these influences are also revealed in the patient narratives examined here. Thus improving clinical services and making them less dehumanizing for patients and physicians requires interventions to change the cultures of health care, especially the health-care bureaucracy and health-care economics.

No doubt partially reflecting the patient's awareness of these forces, a single negative doctor-patient experience is often transferred to the entire clinical facility, to an entire category of clinical programs, or to the entire health-care system. The subsequent reluctance to seek treatment after a negative encounter may function as an enduring barrier to treatment. This phenomenon of transference provides even more incentive for health-care institutions to make treatment less dehumanizing for patients.

Another implication for clinical services has to do with cultural similarity and difference. In view of my interactions with Ashley (the Chinese American patient who preferred not to have an Asian therapist) and my Calabrian patient (who reacted to the similarity implied by my last name), we should pay attention to problematic aspects of cultural similarity as well as cultural difference. We should learn from patients which aspects of similarity they find problematic but remain open to the therapeutic possibilities that working through such difficulties might offer.

Even in an age of new medical technologies and increasingly bureaucratized health-care systems, many patients in the United States are still looking for a traditional doctor-patient relationship. However, technological innovation and economic and bureaucracy-driven changes in the cultures of health care, such as the time limits imposed on meetings with psychiatrists or the privileging of medication over psychotherapy, are creating new models of care that conflict with the treatment expectations of patients. As such, a "clinical paradigm clash" (Calabrese 2008) is at work within the changing structure of U.S. health care between traditional patient expectations and new forms of bureaucratized practice. These paradigm clashes within mainstream health-care systems are as important for anthropological study as the more familiar clashes that occur between mainstream health-care systems and various indigenous systems of diagnosis and treatment (see Fadiman 1997). Both reveal the interplay of cultural interpretations, social structures, and dynamics of power and the impact they have on the relationships between patients and their clinicians.

References

Calabrese, Joseph D. 2008. "Clinical Paradigm Clashes: Ethnocentric and Political Barriers to Native American Efforts at Self-Healing." *Ethos: Journal of the Society for Psychological Anthropology* 36(3): 334–53.

Desjarlais, Robert. 2000. "The Makings of Personhood in a Shelter for People Considered Homeless and Mentally Ill." *Ethos: Journal of the Society for Psychological Anthropology* 27(4): 466–89.

DiGiacomo, Susan M. 1987. "Biomedicine as a Cultural System: An Anthropologist in the Kingdom of the Sick." In *Encounters with Biomedicine: Case Studies in Medical Anthropology*, edited by Hans A. Baer. New York: Gordon and Breach.

Eisenberg, Leon. 1977. "Disease and Illness." *Culture, Medicine and Psychiatry* 1(1): 9–23.

Fadiman, Anne. 1997. *The Spirit Catches You and You Fall Down.* New York: Farrar, Straus and Giroux.

Foucault, Michel. 1973. *The Birth of the Clinic: An Archaeology of Medical Perception.* New York: Vintage Books.

Good, Mary-Jo DelVecchio, and Byron J. Good. 2000. "Clinical Narratives and the Study of Contemporary Doctor-Patient Relationships." In *Handbook of Social Studies in Health and Medicine*, edited by Gary Albrecht, Ray Fitzpatrick, and Susan Scrimshaw. London: Sage Publications.

Good, Mary-Jo DelVecchio, Cara James, Byron J. Good, and Anne E. Becker. 2003. "The Culture of Medicine and Racial, Ethnic, and Class Disparities in Health Care." In *Unequal Treatment: Confronting Racial and Ethnic Disparities in Health Care*, edited by Brian D. Smedley, Adrienne Y. Stith, and Alan Ray Nelson. Washington, D.C.: National Academies Press.

Gray, Bradford H. 1997. "Trust and Trustworthy Care in the Managed Care Era." *Health Affairs* 16(1): 34–49.

Hopper, Kim. 2001. "Commentary: On the Transformation of the Moral Economy of Care." *Culture, Medicine and Psychiatry* 25(4): 473–84.

Jenkins, Janis H., and Elizabeth Carpenter-Song. 2008. "Stigma Despite Recovery: Strategies for Living in the Aftermath of Psychosis." *Medical Anthropology Quarterly* 22(4): 381–409.

——. 2009. "Awareness of Stigma Among Persons with Schizophrenia: Marking the Contexts of Lived Experience." *Journal of Nervous and Mental Disease* 197(7): 520–59.

Keane, Mary. 1990. "Contemporary Beliefs About Mental Illness Among Medical Students: Implications for Education and Practice." *Academic Psychiatry* 14(3): 172–77.

Kirschner, Suzanne R., and William S. Lachicotte. 2001. "Managing Managed Care: Habitus, Hysteresis and the End(s) of Psychotherapy." *Culture, Medicine and Psychiatry* 25(4): 441–56.

Mechanic, David. 1997. "Managed Care as a Target of Distrust." *Journal of the American Medical Association* 277(22): 1810–811.

Rao, Harish, H. Mahadevappa, P. Pillay, M. Sessay, A. Abraham, and J. Luty. 2009. "A Study of Stigmatized Attitudes Towards People with Mental Health Problems Among Health Professionals." *Journal of Psychiatric and Mental Health Nursing* 16(3): 279–84.

Silverman, W. H. 1996. "Cookbooks, Manuals, and Paint-by-Numbers: Psychotherapy in the 90's." *Psychotherapy* 33(2): 207–15.

U.S. Department of Health and Human Services (HHS). 1999. *Mental Health: A Report of the Surgeon General.* Rockville, Md.: Government Printing Office.

Velpry, Livia. 2008. "The Patient's View: Issues of Theory and Practice." *Culture, Medicine and Psychiatry* 32(2): 238–58.

Weber, Max. 1946. *From Max Weber: Essay in Sociology,* trans. by Hans H. Gerth and C. Wright Mills. New York: Oxford University Press.

Yang, Lawrence H., Arthur Kleinman, Bruce G. Link, Jo C. Phelan, Sing Lee, and Byron J. Good. 2007. "Culture and Stigma: Adding Moral Experience to Stigma Theory." *Social Science & Medicine* 64(2007): 1524–535.

Chapter 10

The Paper Life of Minority and Low-Income Patient Care

ANTONIO BULLON, MARY-JO DELVECCHIO GOOD,
AND ELIZABETH CARPENTER-SONG

Instead of documenting what we do, documenting is what we do.
—Psychiatric nurse

I am just a psychiatrist who sees every kind of patient from different ethnic, cultural backgrounds with neuropsychiatric disorders, and also I devote myself to this particular role of treating Latino patients.
—Academic psychiatrist

Medical practice must be regulated, but the form this currently takes is increasingly based on a "technical" view, which wrongly assumes that practice is straightforward and that error is the result of individual failure.
—C. Cole, *Advances in Psychiatric Treatment*

Throughout this book, we explore how a variety of social factors exogenous to clinical medicine, narrowly conceived, are critical mediators of experiences of clinicians and patients and the quality of care. Central to our analysis is an argument about the role of new forms of ethnic diversity, what we have called *hyperdiversity*. However, our investigations found that the culture of medicine that shapes clinician experience and practice is deeply influenced by administrative and financial requirements, as well as by the meaning and values that give distinctive form to American medicine.

We approach our analyses from two vantage points—that of a psychiatrist-researcher (Antonio Bullon)—the ultimate participant observer—and that of anthropologists and observers (Elizabeth Carpenter-Song and Mary-Jo DelVecchio Good) who are distanced from the obligations and demands of clinical life and the moral responsibilities of caring for patients. Our research and analysis from these various stances reveals a portrait of contemporary psychiatry as shaded by uncertainty, fraught with tensions caused by diminished professional control over clinic time induced by a rising technological mode of documentation, paperwork, and legal regulations designed to improve efficiency, and by day-to-day struggles to provide good care to ethnic minorities, new immigrants, and low-income patients in contexts of strictly limited resources (Good et al. 2003). For this essay, we use the terms *psychiatry* or *psychiatric* to reference all mental health disciplines, not only the medical specialty of psychiatry.

The voices from the life worlds of psychiatry, through interviews with clinicians and administrators, and a narrative account of mundane clinical culture by Dr. Bullon, bring us into the trenches of psychiatric care for low-income, mostly Spanish-speaking patients.[1] Challenges that loom large for clinicians in these settings, in addition to the provision of culturally competent care, arise from an astonishing increase in documentation requirements—or paperwork and a checkbox psychiatry—that has replaced narrative-based patient records.[2] Such documentation practices create a parallel paper life for both psychiatrists and patients, a life quite removed from patient life narratives and the clinical realities and experiences of psychiatrists with their patients.

This essay de-centers a mainstream perspective within medicine that emphasizes patient culture as a problem to be addressed, and instead elaborates trends in the cultures of psychiatric practice and health care as problematic. In the opinion of mental health providers interviewed, the enormous increase in documentation and technical rational practices—a salient aspect of the current culture of clinical practice—leads to fragmentation of clinical work, at times compromising the meaningful care of patients and double-binding clinicians. According to these narratives, those most affected by these factors are patients who are poor and belong to minority groups.

We enter the field through a psychiatrist's reflections on mundane practices of daily clinical work at the Latino Clinic that can lead to the fragmentation of patient care. In reading the account, the reader should hear it voiced with ironic humor, high dramatic flourishes, and colored by foxhole laughter (see Luhrmann 2000, 119). This narrative method of reflective practitioners is used in the social and medical sciences to convey an understanding of professional experience. This approach reflects Donald Schon's early influential work on narrative and the professions in *The Reflective Practitioner* (1983), as well as the more recent efforts to promote the use of narrative in medicine by Columbia University physician Rita Charon (2006).[3]

Monday Morning at the Latino Clinic: Reflections of a Psychiatrist

I dread Mondays, but especially Mondays of the past few years. When I arrive at my office in an outpatient psychiatry clinic serving a large number of low income patients, most of whom speak only Spanish, I sigh when I view the two piles of paperwork that lie placidly and intrusively on my desk. They flank a silent phone, which lets me know through its blinking red light that it also has pending business with me. The mounds of papers are mostly forms from various sources. One from the housing authority of a particular town requesting my opinion about one of my patient's diagnoses and the appropriateness of granting him a preferential place on a waiting list for subsidized apartments. Another was dropped by another patient the week before asking for medical information that will determine the need to be entitled to state-subsidized transportation.

I glimpse several unopened envelopes. Because of their familiar pattern on the edges, I am pretty sure these envelopes come from the Social Security Administration and are asking me for clinical details and for my opinion regarding whether a patient of mine is able to return to work or if he is entitled to continue receiving disability benefits.

I know that none of these requests are irrelevant. They all require a medical practitioner's signature. Any delay in filling out these documents could jeopardize the possibility of my patients getting help. In some cases these documents are essential for my patient's survival in this world. Despite this importance, I cannot help feeling frustrated, invaded by a strong sense of absurdity. I feel I shouldn't be spending so much of my time filling out forms and papers.

I decide to check my voice mail. My guess regarding the content of many of the messages left over the weekend turns out to be correct. There are the polite ones with an apologetic tone: "Sorry doctor, I know you are very busy, but those papers are so important." These patients wonder if I have received the papers that they dropped off last week or the week before. Have I filled them out? They have not heard from me. Perhaps they left the messages reminding me at the wrong phone number? Other messages include calls from pharmacies informing me that I need to fill out a "prior authorization" form for certain medications I prescribed to some of my patients. These messages are followed by the anxious and sometimes frantic calls from those patients who are confused and frustrated by what is happening. Many of them have been receiving the same medications for years, but because of changes in medication formularies, they now required "PA." While I am getting a glimpse of what promises to be a "fun paperwork day," I get a page from my secretary: my first patient of the day has arrived.

I greet Juan Rodriguez in the waiting room. He is a very pleasant sixty-year-old Puerto Rican gentleman, whom I have seen for the past four years. He was referred to me by his primary care provider in the midst a psychotic depression. Since then, he has received medications and psychotherapy and he has done extremely well. He is very compliant with the medication regimen I prescribe and goes to see his therapist religiously. Today, he looks unusually concerned. He shows me a list of his medications that my secretary has just given him. When he asked her the reason for that unusual procedure, he was told, "the doctor will explain." Unfortunately, I am also at a loss, but then I remember information that went to a corner in my brain. It had come in a recent email from the hospital's Quality Assurance Committee informing clinicians that after the last JCAHO[4] visit, the hospital was found deficient in the area of medication reconciliation The clinician is required to update the medication list, give it to the patient, and inform the next practitioner whom the patient will see about medication changes. Certainly an excellent effort for improving healthcare quality! No clinicians in their right mind would oppose it . . . ah, but "the time." (Bullon's narration)

Documentation and Paperwork As Clinical Culture in Psychiatric Practice

Over the past two decades, paperwork has taken a predominant place among activities performed by mental health practitioners, affecting the nature of clinical work and the psychiatric record—the patient's record. The most obvious changes in inpatient settings are replacement of the traditional narrative format of clinical notes with predominantly checkbox-based notes and multiplication of regulatory, legal, and patient-rights forms. In outpatient clinics, most notable are standardized language progress notes through template-based formats and an abundance of other forms: treatment plan reviews required by managed care companies for authorization of continued services, applications for prior authorization of certain medications, requests for social services, and a variety of consent forms.

The Paper Life and The Technological Mode

> Instead of documenting what we do, documenting is what we do.
> —Psychiatric nurse

The experiences recounted by the psychiatrist are shared by many other mental health clinicians who find themselves overwhelmed and often annoyed by the demands of paperwork, which they experience as "intrusions from outside," compromising their professional identity. These requirements are in fact major manifestations of important social, political, economic, and historical factors that are present within as well as outside medicine and psychiatry, and the forces that led to the transformations in documentation practices include powerful movements in cost containment, defensive medicine, health-care quality assurance. Many documentation practices are also the legislative fruits of years-long efforts of patient advocacy groups.

The institutionalization of these practices reflect a rise in "the technological mode," (Phillips 2002), a major way of acting and thinking in contemporary medical and psychiatric practice that grows out of the standardization of knowledge and practice, the categorization of problems with matching solutions as exemplified in practice guidelines. Many clinicians—including those we interviewed for this project and those others have interviewed—experience a minimization of the value of professional judgment of individual clinicians (Donald 2001; Good 1995a; Good 1994). In particular, many clinicians are concerned that the technological mode, in emphasizing documentation practices that delete the complexities of patients lives, may be most problematic when caring for minority and poor patients, patients who clinicians professionally refer to as having socially complex problems, but in times of stress may use more emotionally charged and pejorative terms such as *trainwrecks* (Good et al. 2003). A common discourse among clinicians is the complaint that documentation requirements and practices do not account for the intricate decision making process that occurs in the real clinical life of psychiatric practice, and especially—as we will see through several clinical scenarios—the complex realities of caring for disadvantaged patients.

Consent Forms, Legalities, and Patient Rights

Medical services are legally required to offer privacy, confidentiality forms, and patients' rights forms. Outpatient clinics usually present to patients a package with the HIPAA (Health Insurance Portability and Accountability Act) form and several printed papers to consent to receive care in the facility, to bill their insurance companies, or to communicate with other medical providers. Patient-advocacy forces have conditioned the legal requirement for informed consent and privacy protections. For quality assurance organizations, regulatory agencies, and for some hospital administrators, such paperwork is viewed positively, as a tangible record of patient protection and catalyst for patient empowerment:

> The presence of HIPAA consent forms or other patient rights forms is an opportunity to discuss openly what is already implicit in the patient-clinician relationship: the respect for patient individuality, his control over his treatment. It decreases paternalism, especially in vulnerable populations. (Administrator clinician)

Yet, for some patients and their clinicians, consent forms appear to hold little relevance, and in fact may not reflect an advancement in the quality of care and respect to minority or poor patients, as an outpatient psychiatrist notes:

I work with a large population of patients who speak only Spanish. When they are seen for the first time, they are offered the HIPAA agreement, which is presented to them by the secretaries. Although the document is in Spanish, it produces confusion in my poorest and less educated patients, although all of them end up signing the document. I would finally meet with the patients and ask them if they understood what they were signing, most of them would say they did not know. They would tell me, "I trust in you, whatever you think is necessary, doctor."

Whereas physician forms supporting housing or Social Security benefits provide practical results that are no doubt essential from the perspective of patients, consent forms appear to hold little if any instrumental value. Both patients and clinicians often find themselves simply going through the motions of signing consent documents as a legal formality. Moreover, the laborious process of physicians reviewing consent documents may consume precious minutes of an already brief therapeutic encounter. In this vein, an outpatient psychiatrist expresses his frustration:

I have complained to my clinic administrator about the time that it takes to explain to some of my Latino patients what really means the HIPAA. She told me that she thinks it is advancement in patient rights because by explaining their rights and ask them to sign, they may take more responsibility for their treatment and decrease paternalism. Although this concept is good, I don't think I can solve years of disempowerment or social inequalities by having them sign one form. Also, I don't have time to explain the document to all of them either. I trust that I am doing things in good faith and in benefit of the patient, and instead choose to spend time trying to understand what is troubling them.

Parallel Lives: The Paper Life in the Context of Social Chaos

Mental health clinicians attempt to meet what administrators, insurance companies and accreditation agencies are looking for, but in this effort, they may find themselves creating and living parallel lives. This experience is particularly frequent for clinicians who care for poor and minority patients with complicated life situations. One life unfolds in the clinical encounter and the other is the life documented in the chart, what we call the paper life. Providers find that documentation mandates and expectations do not fit the complexities of clinical practice or of patient life. Borrowing a phrase from Christine Ceci (2008), the requirements have become "increasingly distant from life." This dilemma is vividly recounted by a psychiatrist working on the Latino team:

I have followed Mercedes for the past ten years, a Puerto Rican woman in her mid-fifties who suffers from chronic and recurrent major depression, generalized anxiety disorder, and PTSD from childhood neglect and several abusive relationships in the past. She also is dealing with diabetes, osteoarthritis, COPD [chronic obstructive pulmonary disease], and morbid obesity. Her fifth-grade education and limited English allowed her to do several cleaning jobs until a few years ago when she was placed on SSDI [Social Security Disability Insurance] because of her health problems. She lives in an apartment in the projects. Despite multiple combinations of psychotropics, her symptoms have never gone into complete remission. Lately she has been stable, but a few days ago she showed up suddenly in my office, crying, expressing severe insomnia and suicidal thoughts. . . . She had a serious situation with the housing authority because she had not responded to a previous letter asking her to show up with documentation of proof of her current income and bills. I spent part of the session in figuring out what was really happening and referred her to our community resource specialist, a bilingual ancillary staff that could assist her in filling out the form and meeting housing's requirements. At her request to change her medications "because they were not working," I proposed she wait until her current housing crisis had been resolved. If by then the symptoms persisted at such severity, I would consider modifying her regimen.

In fact I have already been concerned about her polypharmacy, a result from my—sometimes desperate—efforts to help her suffering. But by attempting to solve her social chaos with medications originally aimed at treating well defined psychiatric conditions (she met criteria for at least three of them), I was probably also contributing to her serious medical problems. Later that day, when I was writing the progress note for this encounter, I remember the mandatory "coding and documentation compliance seminar" that I attended a few weeks ago, that focused on how "psychiatrists should document for services that reflect the unique interventions that stem from their technical expertise." "Nonmedical" interventions are not reimbursable and they should not be documented as the main part of that intervention. Because my session with Mercedes was a psychopharmacological visit, I had to document that a great part of the session was devoted to assessing and intervening on her symptoms with treatment. If I were to write that in fact, I had used most of the session in exploring social issues that are crucial for my intervention to result in a good clinical outcome, even though this is not part of my unique technical expertise, there is a risk that the session will not be reimbursed.

Many clinicians working with minority and poor patients are faced with the fact that managed care documentation templates do not include critical interventions that must be made at a social dimension. The documentation and record-keeping practices of contemporary clinical life are often experienced by many mental health clinicians as oversimplifications of socially complex and chaotic life realities. In contrast, the realities of the paper life are often viewed as alien to the therapeutic tasks many clinicians continue to try to view as their main professional activity. The paper life may erase the most significant issues bearing on patient illness and care. Such practices, some argue, lead to fragmentation of therapeutic work and clinical narratives (Good et al. 1994; Good et al. 2003; Good 1985; Mattingly and Garro 1994) without significantly contributing to actions directly related to improving their patients' lives. Clinicians also express frustration with requirements to fit complex social dimensions into ultra-reduced checkbox constructs without a complementary official space in the template to record their efforts to integrate different aspects of their patients' lives. The most complex patients, suffering the most social chaos, become in that way invisible.

Despite these challenges, conscientious providers proceed with a deeper and more personalized engagement with the patient, which has little resemblance with the note or treatment plan update that has been made for "the record" (Donald 2001). Other clinicians, viewing the discrepancy of what is demanded and the time and reimbursement limitations, may resort to a particular compensatory practice in which they "do not do more than they are asked."

Changes in the Clinical Chart and Narrative Construction

The psychiatric record has changed. From a depository of information about patients and the clinical thinking process, it has turned into a collection of legal documents, consent forms, insurance information, acknowledgment forms[5] signed by patients' confirming that they have been informed about their rights. With the exception of the initial psychiatric evaluation, there is a conspicuous scarcity of narrative because progress notes consist of preprinted checkbox forms with a few lines for a free narrative. A recent requirement from a regulatory and quality assurance agency dictates that health-care institutions must inquire about patients' cultural preferences and beliefs regarding their health. To meet that stipulation, some hospitals have added a new variable in the patient record template devoted to demographic information. Next to the several choices of ethnicity and religious affiliation, a line reads "cultural beliefs and preferences" and, next to it, two yes-no checkboxes and the word *explain*, followed by a two-inch line.

The use of the checkbox approach may also have important ramifications in the way clinicians see their patients. Byron Good (1994) has elaborated how the practice of writing about the patient in the medical chart is not only a literary representation of the world, but also a powerful way of acting. By forcing themselves to use different interpretations and paradigms, clinicians create new ways of integrating and conceptualizing different aspects of their patients. This is particularly important for patients who belong to social and cultural backgrounds that may be very different from that of the clinician, who may have an initial impulse to increase a sense of certainty by placing the patient in a category familiar to the practitioner. The daily narrative of the events, new information, and new interactions with the patient, along with the evolution of clinical thinking, provide an unique opportunity to accept complexity and uncertainty and—it is hoped—a greater respect for the patient who is "different."

What is the effect of a psychiatric record in which narrative gradually disappears and is replaced by standardized information that does not contribute to understanding all the different worlds and dimensions that affect patients, especially the poorest and most disenfranchised? Clinicians including psychiatric nurses complain that the patient chart "is full of forms that don't help you much" and "that the best way to know what is happening with patients is being present in daily clinical rounds. . . . Everybody involved can say what is of concern." Others report that they have to "keep unofficial notes of their patients, so they can maintain the continuity of what is happening with them." One psychiatric nurse interviewed gave an example of how checkbox documentation may impede patient care by comparing the patient records of the narrative past with the checkbox templates of the present:

> In the past when one of us returned to the unit after being away for a few days, it sufficed to read the other nurses' notes about a particular patient to know how the patient was doing. With the changes in the nurses' notes (to checkbox documentation), we resort to reading the attending process note, but now they also don't have much information. In these days we have to read in many different places to put bits and pieces together to have a sense of what is happening with the patients.

Mental Health Clinicians As Gatekeepers

Even though clinicians from all areas have encountered an explosion in the amount of paperwork, the situation is much more dramatic in clinical work with disadvantaged and minority patients who are likely to present with a constellation of mental health and medical problems as well as social needs. In contemporary society, many social problems have been medicalized, and thus, the clinician working with disenfranchised patients is positioned as gatekeeper to a range of basic services beyond the scope of mental health care. As one clinician in our study observes,

> I have to accept that this is a reality that is part of taking care of these patients. I feel they are forced by a blind system to seek help from doctors. They hear from their family, friends, or neighbors: "If you are having

problems with such and such (basic services and needs) issue, ask your doctor to fill out a letter saying that you are sick." If I were poor, probably I'd do the same thing.

The proper documentation—the right form with the right signature—grants access to needed services for disadvantaged people. An outpatient psychiatrist working with Latino patients told us,

> I feel that three out of five of the patients that I see for psychopharmacological treatment will end up bringing me some type of form to fill out during the course of their treatment. One homeless patient wants to be on a priority list to get housing, while other patients that live in subsidized apartments want to change their place of residence because they live in a dangerous neighborhood. Or it may be that some others want to expedite obtaining transitional assistance because they are jobless and don't have any money, or they want subsidized transportation, etc. . . . All of these requests come with a form to fill.

Often psychiatrists working with poor and needy patients, including ethnic minority or immigrant patients, feel underappreciated and undercompensated; an outpatient psychiatrist remarked, "I don't think the hospital understands very well how difficult and demanding it is to work with poor patients. We physicians have to do a lot of extra work, but we have the same time and productivity expectations as our peers."

For some clinicians, housing and Social Security authorization forms may be but a nuisance or an annoyance, whereas for others this paperwork undermines professional identity, tainting clinical work. A psychiatrist explained his approach:

> I really don't fill out any paperwork unless [patients] are established in their care with me, and I see they are interested in receiving care. . . . I think it is not right to fill in information on somebody you don't know. I am not here to fill out paperwork, I am here to be their doctor. . . . There should be other places dedicated to that. Sometimes I feel that I have stopped being a doctor, and I have become a social worker.

Another clinician remarked, "I understand why patients need to come to me with paperwork, but truthfully, I don't like the situation. I understand it but I feel manipulated."

Frustration, Burnout, and Alienation

Certainly the amount of paperwork that comes with the care of disadvantaged patients is much greater than with patients that belong to higher social status and well-educated groups. There is an overabundance of paperwork that is essential to patients' lives, and clinicians who have chosen the professional path of working with disadvantaged populations cannot ignore it—even if it produces frustration and resentment—if interventions are to be successful. Clinicians lower on the professional hierarchy and younger—the residents and junior attendings and other trainees—are most likely to be the frontline providers for neediest patients, many of whom are poor or from ethnic minorities and have medically, psychiatrically, and socially complex lives. From the perspective of a senior psychiatry attending, young clinicians are more vulnerable to burnout and frustration even though they are committed to serving all patients, particularly the needy. Other clinicians who cannot choose their patients or the type of practice they work in also appear more likely to express frustration, resentment, ambivalence, and alienation with the competing demands of quality patient care, documentation, and social service paperwork. The following interview excerpts with clinicians are illustrative.

Resentment and Ambivalence Toward Patients

Some clinicians perceived certain patients as morally suspect, manipulative agents. As a psychiatry resident said,

> I resent sometimes having to fill out forms after forms that many of my patients bring. Many times I can see an envelope that they carry in the hand even in the first visit, and I wonder to myself: "What will it be this time?" I feel bad for feeling frustrated because I know that probably there is no other way for poor patients to obtain needed benefits. Occasionally I encounter patients that really frustrate me because I believe they are taking advantage of the system . . . even though they are poor, they seem to want everything to be paid for them.

Yet, for patients, a physician's signature is necessary as is paperwork for obtaining resources and services. However, psychiatrists frequently feel that their role as a patient's physician and advocate is compromised by paperwork and requests for disability status, which they experience as "manipulative" and inappropriate.[6]

Another psychiatrist who cares for Latino patients echoes this sentiment: "Sometimes it is impossible not to think that some of these patients are 'milking the system' and that they are only coming to get their paperwork filled out. It is hard not to get angry inside . . . then I see that there are very few other places willing to help them."

Some clinicians fear becoming punitive with their patients. A young psychiatric social worker in a Latino mental health clinic related some changes in her attitudes towards certain patients:

> I am afraid that I have become skeptical with some of my patients. When I started working in this clinic, I was moved by everybody's problems

and needs, but as time has passed by, I have become a little bit cynical with some of them when I suspect that they are trying to take advantage of being sick and being poor. In my supervision, I constantly talk about my fear of becoming punitive towards some patients.

Resentment Toward Administration and Regulatory Agencies

Clinicians in the front line of provision of care to minority and poor patients are also at greatest risk of feeling disconnected from the purpose of the documentation requirements and to perceive them as an imposition from above. Because they have little ownership over the decision-making process, they often feel resentment toward administration, managed care companies, policymakers, and regulatory agencies for "making them do something that does not make sense," that appears to be redundant or unnecessary. Alternatively, they may feel overwhelmed or inadequate by trying to meet—at a high cost of personal time and energy—all the duties expected of a competent and ethical clinician. A senior academic psychiatrist observes this:

> It seems that the people doing the clinical work do not have access to the reasons why important regulations were implemented. On the other hand, the people that implemented these policies have done so with good intentions without realizing the consequences along the way. This is like a puppet show in which puppets do not know why the strings are being pulled, and the puppeteers do not know how the puppet is moving. They are both frustrated with the results. They are not aware of each other. It is a real tragedy.

Following the Rules of the Game

Experienced clinicians working with poor minority patients often develop a more cynical approach, playing the rules of the game and responding in a routine and standardized way to what managed care companies or agencies are looking for; yet they seek to keep the encounter with the patient intact. Clinicians may copy and paste key wording that will be repeated in multiple forms that belong to different patients, only to add a few details pertinent to a particular patient, as described by the attending psychiatrist in an outpatient clinic that serves low-income and minority patients:

> Every number of visits, I have to fill out a treatment plan update for insurance companies, in order to receive authorization of visits. Truthfully, whatever I write there is almost the same for all patients. I know that the

insurance companies only care about certain words regarding presence and severity of symptoms and level of functioning. That is taken care by phrases such as "severe depressive symptoms produce attention and concentration problems and low energy which interfere with patient's work and relationships." In terms of the treatment you have to put something like: "with treatment patient has improved at least 50 percent in his mood, but he is not at his baseline yet." They ask for date of discharge from treatment. That means when you predict the patient will be recovered. I write six to eight months from the date. Most of the time, I don't believe that is the case. In fact, I don't know if they really read what I write.

As noted by a senior outpatient psychiatrist, others know the rules of the game as well.

Pharmaceutical companies instruct the doctors in the use of the 'magic words' that will open the door to "prior authorization" medication approval. I'm sure that insurance companies are aware of this game, so it is evident to me that the way they are trying to cut costs is not through a 'rational clinical decision process' but through the implementation of absurd and time-consuming requirements that will discourage the clinician to prescribe the restricted medication.

Conclusion

As this chapter illustrates, many clinicians experience documentation practices and the paper life as frustrating and problematic, particularly when taking care of patients with complex problems or from diverse backgrounds. However, psychiatry has accepted the documentation templates and checkboxes, as well as best practice guidelines and algorithmic approaches, as being useful and even life-saving in certain situations.[7] Yet, a narrow application of the idea that every problem in medicine is a technologically solvable dilemma, without consideration for social complexities and the life world of patients, has caused unintended consequences of fragmentation. Paradoxically, this approach may not achieve the intended goals of improving care and, in fact, may worsen the quality of patient care. Some of these measures may accentuate disparities in health care in the most vulnerable populations, the poor disadvantaged minorities, with complex psychiatric and medical conditions and with socially chaotic lives, who defy the goals of a modeled care that provides rapid assessment and efficient treatment (Good et al. 2003, 602).

The technological mode and its underlying mentality create parallel lives: the one that occurs in the clinical encounter and the other that is documented in the chart or in other forms of the paper life, such as the increasingly widespread electronic medical record (Hartzband and

Groopman 2008). The mismatch between a set of inflexible documentation demands and the complexity of clinical reality forces clinicians to live in a duplicitous world, in which they have to learn new skills in wording phrases that meet official requirements but have little resemblance to actual clinical encounters.

If ethnic and racial disparities in health status and health care stem from multidimensional processes (Good et al. 2003, 597), simple and nominal approaches such as the signature on a consent form, or the mark in checkbox on an intake form in the psychiatric record confirming that patient was asked about religious preferences, health-care beliefs, or ethnic identity, will not necessarily reflect that a medical institution or a psychiatric clinician is devoted to take into account patients' cultural explanations or fears about their illness. Will the technological mode of documentation and best practice guidelines help to reduce health-care disparities with certain minorities? It is unclear. Checkbox and documentation practices may at times give a false cosmetic reassurance to the medical institution, to providers, to the regulatory agencies, and to society in general, and imply that issues regarding inequalities in care with people from minorities who are poor have been addressed. This illusion may preclude closer examination of the cultures of psychiatric practices, its institutions of care, and its providers, and how these may impede the provision of culturally sensitive, high-quality, and equitable care. If clinicians become alienated from the medical systems in which they practice in response to the disconnection between mandated documentation and paperwork and their own clinical realities, they may develop resentment toward the very patients who require extra effort and time and are not easy to treat. They may opt out of caring for these more difficult populations, thus reproducing disparities in care for minorities and disadvantaged patients.

A Coda: Recommendations

It would be ironic to offer technical recommendations to approach the double life created by a set of formulaic interventions that are not congruent with the real clinical life. Interventions must occur at different levels where pressures, such as cost containment, influence the values and actions of the culture of medicine and transform very complex realities into oversimplified constructs. The following recommendations are proposed to improve quality of care in particular for minority and disadvantaged patients.

At the societal level, there must be open discussion of how narrowly applied technological solutions may not yield the efficacy and efficiency that are sought by all stakeholders, including the cost-containment agencies themselves. Systematic qualitative and quantitative research is needed to determine the extent to which the degree of burnout among younger frontline providers negatively affects clinical outcomes, or the extent to which the drive for efficacy leads to harm due to isolated psychopharmacological interventions for complex and disadvantaged populations.

Clinical educators—the medical faculty and clinical administrators—should constantly emphasize that diagnostic guidelines, checklists, and protocols should be used as tools to enhance the therapeutic alliance, but should not replace it. Pressures from reimbursement and regulatory agencies that are contradictory to the goals of enhancing quality of care should be openly discussed in individual supervision and public clinical forums without concern for retaliation. Managed care companies and quality assurance and accrediting agencies should encourage clinician feedback in open sessions in which these agencies, administrators, and clinicians discuss the rationale behind documentation modalities and requirements, and receive recommendations from clinicians. This will help shape the tools of the documentary mode to better fit clinical reality and ultimately improve quality of care.

Clinical centers and managed care companies must provide additional compensated time or allocate support staff to meet certain quality improvement requirements—such as medication reconciliations—in order to avoid relying on the already strained clinician's regular schedule. In addition, there should be compensation for the extra time required to ascertain complex social realities of poor and minority patients?

Another way that clinical centers and managed care companies should show their commitment to fostering the rights of disadvantaged patients is by recruiting and financially supporting services of culturally competent ancillary staff who act as health-care navigators in the complex medical system for minorities who are not proficient in English, are poor, have little education, or have complex psychiatric and medical problems.

Additionally, medical centers should conduct ongoing educational and empowerment seminars for patients and their families through support groups, role playing sessions, and informational lectures to help them better understand and recognize what happens in the medical encounter, what their clinicians' expectations are, and how they may enhance their ability to communicate and have their needs met.

Notes

1. Clinicians interviewed (by Antonio Bullon) belonged to several mental health disciplines and were involved in different types of practice, with different responsibilities and levels of seniority. Those interviewed included psychiatric residents, attending psychiatrists, clinical psychologists, and nurses working in ambulatory clinics (in general psychiatry outpatient clinics and in a mental health clinic devoted to Latino patients), on inpatient

services, and in private practices. Whereas most were involved in direct patient care, some had the added responsibility of case management and administration of clinical services. A few were also active in academic and teaching activities.

2. Joel Braslow, unpublished manuscript delivered to a workshop on Pharmaceutical Selves, convened by Janis Jenkins (2011), School of American Research, Santa Fe, October 2007, in which Mary-Jo DelVecchio Good was also a participant. Braslow compared psychiatric records of today (checkbox) with the lengthy narrative form of psychiatric records from the 1950s to the 1980s documenting the gradual elimination of narrative components in official records (personal communication). See also Gardiner Harris, "Talk Doesn't Pay, So Psychiatry Turns Instead to Drug Therapy," *New York Times*, March 6, 2011.

3. Narrative analysis in medical anthropology has long been a prominent mode of interpretation and method. These efforts are grounded in a vast literature on physician narratives, clinical narratives, therapeutic narratives, illness narratives, and narratives in medicine (Good 1985, 1995a, 1995b; Good 1994; Good and Good 1994; Good et al. 1994; Mattingly and Garro 1994, 2000; Mattingly 1994, 1998; Kleinman 1988).

4. Joint Commission on Accreditation of Health Care Organizations, now simply the Joint Commission.

5. Templates for documentation acknowledging treatments and other clinical actions.

6. A decade earlier a psychiatrist exclaimed similar distress "when patients would ask for disability papers when I thought they should have a job and structure; when I had to turn in many patients for abusing their children; I felt I was in an adversarial role that I did not want to be. Court papers, reports, and people needed social interventions and no one was offering it . . . in the past clinicians had the luxury of time to do paperwork, now they are scheduling brief therapeutic sessions instead of 50 minute sessions to allow time for . . . paperwork" (Good et al. 2003, 602).

7. Gawande makes compelling arguments for the use of checklists in complex medical situations that deal with multiple and concrete variables such as surgical interventions; however this modality does not apply to aspects of clinical care that rely mainly on the human interaction (2009).

References

Ceci, Christine. 2008. "Increasingly Distant from Life: Problem Setting in the Organization of Home Care." *Nursing Philosophy* 9(1): 19–31.

Charon, Rita. 2006. *Narrative Medicine: Honoring the Stories of Illness.* New York: Oxford University Press.

Donald, Alastair. 2001. "The Wal-Marting Of American Psychiatry: An Ethnography of Psychiatric Practice in the Late 20th Century." *Culture, Medicine and Psychiatry* 25(4): 427–39.

Gawande, Atul. 2009. *The Checklist Manifesto: How to Get Things Right.* New York: Henry Holt.

Good, Byron J. 1994. *Medicine, Rationality and Experience: An Anthropological Perspective*. Cambridge: Cambridge University Press.

Good, Byron J., and Mary-Jo DelVecchio Good. 1994. "In the Subjunctive Mode: Epilepsy Narratives in Turkey." *Social Science & Medicine* 38(6): 835–42.

Good, Mary-Jo DelVecchio. 1985. "Discourses on Physician Competence." In *Physicians of Western Medicine*, edited by Robert Hahn and Atwood Gaines. Dordrecht, Neth.: Reidel Publishing.

———. 1995a. *American Medicine: The Quest for Competence*. Berkeley: University of California Press.

———. 1995b. "Cultural Studies of Biomedicine: An Agenda for Research." *Social Science & Medicine* 41(4): 461–73.

———. 2001. "The Biotechnical Embrace." *Culture, Medicine and Psychiatry* 25(4): 385–410.

Good, Mary-Jo DelVecchio, Cara James, Anne Becker, and Byron J. Good. 2003. "The Culture of Medicine and Racial, Ethnic, and Class Disparities in Healthcare." In *Unequal Treatment*, edited by Brian D. Smedley, Adrienne Y. Stith, and Alan Ray Nelson. Washington, D.C.: National Academies Press.

Good, Mary-Jo DelVecchio, Tseunetsugu Munakata, Yasuki Kobayashi, Cheryl Mattingly, and Byron J. Good. 1994. "Oncology and Narrative Time." *Social Science & Medicine* 38(6): 855–62.

Hartzband, Pamela, and Jerome Groopman. 2008. "Off the Record—Avoiding the Pitfalls of Going Electronic." *New England Journal of Medicine* 358(16): 1656–658.

Jenkins, Janis. 2011. *Pharmaceutical Self*. Santa Fe, N.M.: SAR Press.

Kleinman, Arthur. 1988. *The Illness Narratives*. New York: Basic Books.

Luhrmann, Tanya M. 2000. *Of Two Minds*. New York: Alfred A. Knopf.

Mattingly, Cheryl. 1994. "The Concept of Therapeutic Employment." *Social Science & Medicine* 38(6): 811–22.

———. 1998. *Healing Dramas and Clinical Plots*. Cambridge: Cambridge University Press.

Mattingly, Cheryl, and Linda Garro, eds. 1994. "Introduction: Narrative Representations of Illness and Healing," Special issue. *Social Science & Medicine* 38(6): 771–74.

———. 2000. *Narrative and the Cultural Construction of Illness and Healing*. Berkeley: University of California Press.

Phillips, James. 2002. "Managed Care's Reconstruction of Human Existence: The Triumph of Technical Reason." *Theoretical Medicine* 23(4–5): 339–58.

Schon, Donald. 1983. *The Reflective Practitioner*. New York: Basic Books.

Chapter 11

Physicians' Perspectives on Financial Barriers to Equitable Care

SETH DONAL HANNAH, LAWRENCE TAESENG PARK,
AND MARY-JO DELVECCHIO GOOD

THE CHAPTERS in this volume have focused on the role of culture in the process of delivering and accessing health care. However, cultural dynamics play out in the larger context of an evolving system of health-care finance and insurance that powerfully conditions the equitable provision of care. Although equal access to health care is considered by some a fundamental right of citizenship, access to care significantly varies between racial and ethnic groups and between individuals with different levels of income and education.[1]

During the five years we were in the field for this study, major political battles were waged at the national, state, and local levels to expand health insurance and access to health care—first with the landmark 2006 Massachusetts Health Reform Law (referred to in short as Chapter 58) and three years later, with President Barack Obama's similarly structured Patient Protection and Affordable Care Act (ACA).[2] We had the unique opportunity to be in the field as these efforts were debated, enacted, and implemented. Researchers conducted ethnographic observation in the psychiatric inpatient unit and psychiatric emergency department at Academic Medical Center 1[3] in the summer and fall of 2007, and interviewed eight key directors of psychiatric clinics, health-care networks, and emergency rooms in the greater Boston area as well as clinical and support staff. We asked what impact these efforts had on the way they provided care, what barriers continue to limit their patients' access to care, and what they do in their daily work to overcome these barriers.

Clinicians provided detailed accounts of their difficulty navigating the financial system to provide care, but also expressed strong commitment to principles of equity in the provision of care, high levels of frustration over the inadequacy of the system, and striking resilience in crafting novel strategies to subvert bureaucratic hurdles to better take care of their patients. These stories resonate with *Emptying Beds*, Lorna Rhodes' classic ethnography of a psychiatric emergency department, written in 1991 on the heels of another era of tumultuous change in the field of psychiatry, where she found staff in a bind by the mental health system and the institution of care in their attempt to aid severely ill patients. A female psychologist at Academic Medical Center 1 described to us her own attempt at "emptying beds," which was an all too common example of how clinicians in our study attempted to free patients who were "stuck" in the bureaucratic morass of health-care finance and insurance:

> I started calling all the Boston hospitals and they didn't have a bed for free care, for a male. So I started calling a little farther out, and farther out, and farther out, and farther out. Finally I get to a hospital about two and a half hours away, Providence Hospital in Massachusetts, and they pointed out to me that "this is Providence Hospital in Massachusetts, not Providence, Rhode Island. Why are you calling us?" And I said, "There's just no beds available at all. I'm just looking to see if I can find this person some place to go." And they said, "Well, you need to call your congressman about that. . . . We don't have a bed."

Other clinicians told similar stories of how access to certain types of care, particularly mental health care, is severely limited by whether one has insurance and what type of insurance one has. In the case just mentioned, the patient being treated in the psychiatric emergency department was uninsured but became eligible for Free Care, Massachusetts' safety-net insurance program before Chapter 58 was implemented in late 2007.[4] His psychologist decided that he desperately needed to be admitted to an inpatient unit for substance-abuse detox, but no units in a two-and-a-half-hour radius could find room for a patient with this type of insurance, or lack of it. As noted in chapter 10, the insurance status of the patients significantly constrains clinical decision-making. As a female psychiatry resident at Academic Medical Center 2 told us, "It's like a multi-tiered situation and it makes me so angry, because you have to think about finances in your clinical decisions, and I think it's wrong. I mean, you're supposed to [pause] think purely clinically, but you can't. There's a lot of business involved."

Getting Churned

It's certainly the case that access to insurance is huge these days in terms of care. And I'm not all that clear on how the governor's plan to expand access will actually play out. But I think that's a huge factor in determining who gets what and the kind of insurance that you have as well. . . . There's so many people without any insurance and lots of people on Mass Health. And lots of people who then are working and lose their eligibility for Mass Health and become uninsured. And I think those are big factors. I think that they're factors in terms of what you can get access to initially in terms of care, but I think they're also really important in disrupting the continuity of care. When somebody loses insurance and has to change providers, then there goes your therapeutic alliance.

—Female psychiatrist, Academic Medical Center

Clinicians in our study voiced their anxiety over the constantly changing insurance status of their patients. From visit to visit, it is often difficult to know which type of coverage any given patient may have. For three months out of the year a patient may have Mass Health, then after a slight raise in their salary are no longer eligible and have to purchase subsidized insurance through the Commonwealth Connector. If a patient's income decreases he may cycle off of insurance all together for a time, leaving him with no access to care until he can once again afford the premiums for Commonwealth Care. Furthermore, Medicaid and Commonwealth Care have different rules for when eligibility starts and stops, leading to gaps in coverage when transitioning from plan to plan. Coverage can also end for procedural reasons, like when a form documenting income is not returned in time (Dorn, Hill, and Hogan 2009). With each change in insurance status, the process for obtaining prior authorization, different medications eligible for coverage, and different options for referral for aftercare or hospitalization changes. We refer to this phenomenon as "churning" (see also Brandon, Sundaram, and Dunham 2009).

This is particularly problematic for psychiatric care, where name-brand medications are often imperfect substitutes for generics and older medications may be less effective and have more side effects than newer medications. Additionally, fewer treatment centers exist for psychiatric care, and the consequences to discontinuity of care can include immediate safety risks to the patients themselves and to others. A female psychiatrist at Academic Medical Center 1 captured this well when discussing what happens when the insurance status of her patients' changes and she is confronted with an entirely new set of rules about what will be covered:

Well it's a big stress, because you find yourself on the phone for hours and then find yourself up against a stone wall. They can't get the medicine that

you've been giving them for years because . . . it's just terrible. There are
people who have panic attacks, they need to have this.

Clinicians constantly have to adjust their clinical approach due to the
instability of insurance coverage of their patients, threatening their ability to treat their patients according to their own professional clinical
judgment.

Federal public insurance programs such as Medicaid and Medicare
and state-based health-care reforms designed to further expand access
to health insurance, such as Chapter 58 and the ACA, share a common
approach to health-care policy; they all provide tax-funded financing to
pay for private provision of health care. Unlike the National Health
Service in the United Kingdom, the United States, with the exception of
the Veterans Administration (VA) health system, is not involved in
direct provision of health care. Instead, they use public money to either
pay for government-run health insurance programs that pay for care
provided by a network of private hospitals and clinics—Medicaid/Mass
Health and Medicare—or provide cash subsidies for individuals to purchase health insurance from private companies: Commonwealth Care
in Massachusetts and similar "exchange"-based plans under the ACA
starting in 2014. This private-public approach is meant to extend health
insurance coverage to as many people as possible without disrupting the
fundamental market-based structure of American health care—achieving
near-universal coverage.

Our interviews shed light on the effectiveness of this approach on a
national level based on the Massachusetts experience. Studies show that
the number of uninsured nonelderly adults in the Commonwealth
dropped from 12.5 percent in fall 2006—just prior to reform—to 4.8 percent of nonelderly adults in fall 2009 (Long and Stockley 2010). Reform
reduced the number of uninsured by nearly 62 percent, yet according to
the clinicians in our study, the newly insured do not represent a stable
and coherent group of individuals. Instead, the uninsured are perhaps
better viewed as an aggregate measure of the number of uninsured individuals at any given time, with individuals cycling on and off care
according to their particular experience. Interviews conducted by the
Kaiser Family Foundation in 2009 found similar results from the perspective of patients; system complexities can lead to gaps in coverage.
Given the multitude of programs offered by Massachusetts, all with
varying eligibility and programmatic rules, residents with fluctuating
incomes and employment statuses can fall through the cracks. These
individuals, and those who are ineligible for existing programs, still rely
on a health safety net to pay for needed care (Pryor and Cohen 2009).

The clinicians in our study echoed these findings, calling attention
to the disparities in the access to care they experience as a result of

churning. A female psychiatrist at Academic Medical Center explained it this way:

> If there were ways to promote more continuity in care that would be really important in reducing disparities. I think when people have to start over and start anew all the time, a new doctor, a new treatment system, a new provider, that that negatively impacts care. And I think that happens more when people don't have stable employment and stable insurance. I think certainly in terms of economic groups there's disparities related to turnover in insurance and access. As far as clinical cases, there are patients that I've seen who have lost their insurance who then have to be referred to other clinics that take free care or things like that.

The shortfalls revealed by the problem of churning and the continuing difficulties clinicians have providing clinically appropriate care to patients with unstable attachment to the insurance market highlight the distinct difference between the availability of health insurance and actual access to care. Clinicians we interviewed recognized this distinction all too well, and devised strategies to work around the requirements of health insurance and provide needed care to their patients.

Many of these work-arounds took place at the community health centers in our study. Community health-care centers, with patchwork funding from public and private sources, have provided local access to excellent medical care and social services for forty years. In fact, the community health center model originated in Massachusetts with the Columbia Point health center in South Boston in 1965. For patients without private insurance or a public source of payment, they have served as a safety net, providing comprehensive care to anyone in need regardless of their ability to pay through the free care or uncompensated pool system (Hunt 2005). They are typically able to handle commonly seen disorders, but may refer to more specialized facilities, governmental or private, for high levels of care.[5]

The robustness of the free-care system and the strength of community health centers are challenged by the Chapter 58 reforms. Before reform, providers at community health centers would liberally use the free-care system to obtain the care their patients needed without the authorization hassles and close management by private health insurance or the private companies contracted by Medicaid to manage care. The reforms were designed in part to transform this system and provide financially vulnerable populations affordable access to regular health insurance. Patients who were formerly in the free-care system were to be transitioned to public insurance programs such as Mass Health or the new government-subsidized private plans found through the Commonwealth Connector insurance marketplace.

As more people became eligible for Mass Health or purchased plans through the Connector, the funding available for free care at community health centers and designated safety net hospitals would be reduced by concomitant amounts. Recent data on the implementation of health reform in Massachusetts shows that volume and payment of Uncompensated Care Pool/Health Safety Net declined 40 percent from 2007 through the end of 2009. During that period, 408,000 individuals were newly insured, 43 percent going to Commonwealth Care, 24 percent to Mass Health, and 32 percent to group and individual private insurance (Massachusetts Division of Health Care Finance and Policy 2010; Weismann and Bigby 2009). This represents a 36 percent decrease in money for uncompensated care from $656 million in fiscal year 2006 to $417 million in fiscal year 2009. However, some safety net hospitals in Massachusetts contend that volume has not gone down by 40 percent, yet their disproportionate share reimbursements have been cut based on the average rate, not changes in their own payer mix. Boston Medical Center (BMC), the state's largest safety net hospital, filed suit against the state in July 2009 over the issue, alleging the new payment formulas do not cover their reasonable costs (Parmet 2009). Safety net providers are under great pressure to continue to care for a large uninsured population, a good proportion of whom are temporarily or permanently ineligible for state-based insurance (see also Cunningham, Bazzoli, and Katz 2008; Grogan and Gusmano 2009).

Community health centers located in immigrant gateway communities with large numbers of noncitizens in need of care are hit especially hard by these changes (Hunter and Park 2010). At one of our field sites, a community health center located in a diverse low-income urban area north of Boston, clinicians deeply internalized the center's efforts to provide top-quality care for all patients, regardless of their ability to pay, and to provide a variety of social and community services to help smooth their transition to American life. Noncitizens do not qualify for Mass Health or Commonwealth Care under Chapter 58, but are often provided treatment as uninsured patients in the free care–health safety net pool. Although the design of Chapter 58 calls for frontline clinicians to make every effort to find public or private insurance for their patients to minimize the size of the uncompensated pool, this would require asking all patients about their citizenship status and requesting multiple forms of documentation to prove income and employment.

This provides clinicians a difficult choice: move patients onto Mass Health or Commonwealth Care, where they will be confronted with a maze of bureaucratic authorization and managed care—even when doing so may drive away patients from seeking care if they fear deportation—or avoid asking patients about immigration status and directly provide care through the free-care pool.

This can be seen in our conversations with the director of community services:

Q: What are some of the ways that you deal with that or even become aware of somebody's status? How do you deal with that?

Director: Oh gosh, it's just so—it's almost just so second [nature]—I mean it's not even an issue to know about it. It feels like almost everybody we work with in the community health team is undocumented unless they're a refugee, a formalized refugee.

Q: So you just pretty much assume it until you hear otherwise?

Director: Well, um, or it's kind of not an issue . . . we try our best to get patients hooked up with health care if they're available.

Q: Well mechanically, how does that work if there are such widespread undocumented patients, how are they getting care?

Director: The free care. Through the free-care pool. So they get registered for free care.

Q: And that is something that is legitimate?

Director: Is it legitimate? Yeah, it's one of the things, it's just not really asked about at here at least. The free-care pool is huge, the undocumented patients are huge and it's just you know, not even an issue. It's an issue because you're eligible for less. So, when you talk about referring people out or helping them with food stamps, you know things that would really help their well being, then it becomes a big issue.

This exchange shows that the director is comfortable looking away and sidestepping the documentation requirements if it means getting patients the care they need within her health center. Once patients leave the center or try to obtain other benefits, she has less control. It shows a remarkable commitment to providing equitable care and willingness to find cracks in the system to accomplish her goal. Yet the director's approach to working the old free-care system was also dogged by concerns about churning. I asked her about the technical rules regarding citizenship and eligibility and she responded,

> The rules are constantly changing. All I know is that [our health center] sees a huge number of patients that are undocumented and they're all getting free care whether they're getting the limited free care or a version of free care, they're still getting care. So, nobody's not getting care. They might not have great coverage, but nobody's not getting care.

Getting Stuck

During our field work at Academic Medical Center 1, we observed in great detail how clinicians went to battle for their patients in an effort to secure prior authorizations from insurance companies and appropriate referrals and after-care placements throughout the ecology of care in Greater Boston.

The places where coverage issues most often came to a head was in the emergency department and the acute psychiatric inpatient unit. When psychiatric clinicians had to deal with insurance issues, they became indignant. This was true regardless of whether a patient had insurance; in fact, it was probably truer when patients had coverage that was actively managed. We witnessed many frustrated diatribes during our time on the wards, including one that particularly captured the zeitgeist. A female psychiatry resident on the inpatient unit opens by describing the experience of finding an inpatient bed for a substance abuse patient who presented in the emergency department:

> Most people know that like any emergency room these days is kind of a nightmare. You're not an acute patient, so you can sit sometimes six to ten hours waiting to be seen, waiting to get your labs done, and you're already starting to go into withdrawal, feeling terrible, so you're going to leave you know. Just by the function of getting people get medical clearance, probably 50 to 60 percent of the people don't bother, or don't want to have to go through that. And maybe you could say that's weeding out the people who aren't really dedicated to actually getting the detox but I think that that's kind of unfair! They [insurance companies] also say it's important that people get medical clearance before getting detox because what if something's going on? I think that most of the primary physicians could make that decision. A twenty-five-year-old person that doesn't have a lot of medical problems probably doesn't need to get medical clearance before going in for alcohol detox versus a sixty-year-old person with heart disease and you know having had a kidney problem or whatever. They do.

Clinicians feel they have the clinical expertise and have done the necessary face-to-face evaluation. They become frustrated when they have to telephone an insurance representative to secure the care for the patient that they feel is appropriate. In their eyes, the insurance reviewer has not evaluated the patient, and often does not have the qualifications of the clinician. This process amounts to a doctor having to justify admitting a patient to a social worker with a bachelor's or master's degree. Clinicians feel that it is a waste of time and that their clinical judgment is being questioned. The resident just quoted continues:

> The insurance companies . . . just unilaterally make that decision for everybody instead of giving us the freedom to use our clinical skills to decide who should go and who shouldn't. So we're not really the gatekeeper. They're the gatekeeper. And we're the ones kind of trying to like break down the walls to be able to let people get access to the treatment that they need. And it's a really, um, it's a really difficult thing to manage.

Depending on the insurance coverage, it may take several hours to obtain an insurance authorization for the next level of care for this type of patient. On occasion, the insurance reviewer will deny authorization for the recommended level of care—often inpatient level of care, which is the most expensive. In this case, the clinician would need to make an appeal to the reviewer's supervisor. Often the denial of coverage will be upheld by the supervisor. In these cases, the patient may need to be held in the emergency department if it is unsafe to discharge them. In fact, when reviews become contentious, on more than one occasion, reviewers have said that clinicians are free to manage the case whatever way they see fit, but the insurance simply won't pay for the care. In this case, the patient often remains in the emergency department for an extended period because care providers will not accept a referral unless the insurance company has pre-approved the case. The vast majority of patients are unable to cover the costs of an inpatient stay without insurance and end up "stuck" without access to care, even though they had insurance and their treatment was clinically indicated.

As a result of this situation, what often develops is collusion between patient and treater against the insurance company. Although blatant lying is probably too strong a description, both patient and treater have been conditioned to emphasize the safety risk of the clinical presentation. The worst, according to clinicians at Academic Medical Center 1, is Mass Health, the Commonwealth's name for Medicaid. The Commonwealth has subcontracted mental health and substance abuse to private, for-profit insurance companies who have submitted the lowest bid for the contract. In turn, their management of the mental health benefits is such that it is very difficult to get authorization for just about any level of care, and ongoing reviews are conducted frequently, often on a daily basis, with a lot of pressure on the next level of care, usually inpatient, to discharge the patient as soon as possible.

Clinicians feel that it is not only a personal inconvenience for them to go to war with insurance companies, but also that they often desperately need additional time with the patient to make a diagnosis or treatment plan, or to conclude whether they are stable enough to discharge safely into the community. A psychiatry resident discussed how managed care affects her clinical work, saying,

> I think that [managed care] does factor in in terms of things like limitations on the length of inpatient hospital stays. So shorter hospital stays, less time to, you know, get the information that you would want. Less time to discuss the interventions that you would like to do. Less time to think with patients about how they can come to a decision that they're comfortable with. So I think there certainly is a factor that comes from financing and insurance.

Often insurance will only cover certain levels of care, for example, inpatient or outpatient. There may be an alternative level—day treatment, residential treatment, dual diagnosis treatment, assertive community treatment, and so on—that is not covered, and therefore a need to refer to a higher and more expensive level of care. This places clinicians in a bind; patients who they feel are ready for discharge or referral to next-level care get stuck waiting for medication authorizations and coverage for hospitalizations, and other patients are forced out of treatment before they are ready.

Getting Dumped

These problems are even more pronounced when patients do not have insurance, and are either classified as self-pay or Health Safety Net (formerly free care). If a patient is classified as Health Safety Net, they have applied for and been approved for some coverage. Generally speaking, the providing institution will only be compensated for a portion of the care provided; for example, Academic Medical Center 1 gets only 39 percent of the Mass Health negotiated rate for services. The self-pay category is seen by providers as an oxymoron because this group of people have no insurance and no coverage under Health Safety Net—that is, they have no coverage whatsoever. Moreover, these patients will not self-pay for any services.

Managers frequently told us that frontline clinicians often do not understand day-to-day details of the financial standing of their unit. Because there is no compensation for services provided to self-pay patients, the clinicians have mixed feelings about these patients. First, everyone on the treatment side realizes that treatment given to this population of patients will not be compensated. On the other hand, access to emergency and inpatient service for this group of patients is not managed, so clinicians will not have to argue with any reviewers for authorization of any future services. Although not having to get approval lightens the load of the clinician, it is a financial burden on the service. Additionally, particularly for inpatient services, arranging ongoing outpatient care or follow-up services on discharge is difficult. In the emergency department, when patients without insurance present and require hospitalization, mechanisms are in place to contact all hospitals in the Boston area. With the exception of a suburban hospital that is part of Cambridge Health Alliance, Academic Medical Center 1 clinicians know that no other mental health facilities will regularly take uninsured patients. When this occurs, the only viable referral option left is Academic Medical Center 1's own inpatient psychiatry unit. This unit takes a significant share of the uninsured population, but cannot take all uninsured patients: the unit is small for a general hospital of 850 beds, the unit occupancy is almost always at 100 percent, and the unit specializes in medical psychiatric issues and cannot accommodate all the referrals made to the unit.

Still, the refusal to take uninsured patients leads to significant friction between emergency and inpatient staff. Inpatient staff feels that the emergency department is "dumping" on them—another patient for whom there will be no payment—and that arranging aftercare will be difficult. The inpatient staff also realizes that the hospital financial services office is proactive in helping sign up uninsured patients with the appropriate care, usually Mass Health or Health Safety Net, either as approved or pending. In the end, this helps arrange follow-up service.

The emergency department staff, on the other hand, feels that the inpatient staff does not understand the amount of pressure that is on them, and essentially cherry picks to admit the good paying customers. Overall though, when the situation is not acute, most acknowledge that both units of the hospital do more than their fair share in caring for uninsured patients, and other area institutions are not pulling their weight.

This is particularly true of institutions within their hospital network, because there is a feeling that the relationship between institutions should warrant special consideration in accepting uninsured patients but often does not. Clinicians in the emergency department would like to rely on satellite clinics and community health centers, some of which are disproportionate-share providers that get reimbursed at higher rates, that are part of their hospital network to accept referrals and placements because they are often closer to patients' homes and provide a variety of ancillary community-based services. Another feeling that is rarely vocalized but still present is that the uninsured really do not deserve treatment on the inpatient unit, which staff members generally consider to be the best care on the planet. There is a sense of elitism in that the care provided at Academic Medical Center 1 is the best and should be reserved for the worthy.

The relationship between Academic Medical Center and its satellite clinics is also strained by battles over culturally sensitive care, particularly the provision of care in languages other than English. Patients also can get stuck when appropriate clinical services, such as inpatient services, drug rehabilitation, and partial hospital programs, are not available anywhere in the ecology of care.

One of the most common barriers to care that our respondents mentioned was that ethnic minorities and immigrants, in their experience, were more likely to have low income, less likely to have private health insurance, more likely to rely on government health insurance programs, and more likely to be uninsured. Low-income patients without access to good quality insurance are disproportionately found among racial-ethnic minorities and recent immigrants, many of whom live in isolated communities disconnected from flagship hospitals, are not U.S. citizens or legal residents, and do not speak fluent English. In the 1970s, Academic Medical Center 1 began to expand care into these communities, and set up rich community health centers well equipped to handle the diverse language, cultural, and social needs of the residents.

These clinics, however, do not have the capacity to handle all the health-care needs of these patients, and are largely used as feeder sites to bring high-margin business to the flagship hospitals in the city center. This sets up a conflict between investing money to create culturally sensitive outposts in gateway communities and investing in the expansion of culturally sensitive care in Academic Medical Center as well. This conflict bred resentment between clinicians at Academic Medical Center 1, who felt the satellite clinics should be more open to accepting their patients with language and cultural needs, and clinicians at Community Health Center, who felt that clinicians were dumping their nonpaying non-English-speaking, immigrant, and racial-ethnic minority patients on them instead of developing the appropriate capacity themselves.

From the perspective of Academic Medical Center 1 clinicians, they are merely seeking out the best available treatment option for their patients. For example, the director of the Academic Medical Center 1 emergency department gave the following account of her decision-making process when we asked how she takes culture into account when providing treatment. She considers factors such as language, issues of stigma and trust, resistance to treatment, and reliance on alternative healers as part of her options for disposition:

> I want to make a plan for this person to go to the community health center, but does that community center have translators available? Are we putting a plan in place that will ultimately fail? For patients who are Chinese-speaking, we try to refer them to New England Medical Center because they have a very extensive . . . they're in the middle of Chinatown, and they have much more resources in terms of Chinese-speaking staff and other connections to the Chinese community that we just don't have access to here. So we try to draw on the resources that we know about and put those into place. We don't think about the ethnic piece of it. I mean, everybody in America is an immigrant at some level. But when some Italian guy from Revere comes in whose family has lived here for 150 years . . . I'm not going to be thinking about his Italian roots in the same way that it would impact, except for the mafia.

She says she doesn't think of the ethnic piece of it, at least for an Italian mafia member from Revere, yet looks to community centers to provide culturally based care for Chinese-speaking patients, all with the best intentions.

Clinicians and managers at Community Health Center see it from the other side of the coin. Their mental health services were so overcrowded that the continued referral of patients for their top-flight brand of cultural care was stretching them to the breaking point, eventually forcing them to limit access to their outpatient mental health service to individuals with primary care providers at the center—blocking all new referrals from Academic Medical Center 1 and other primary care clinics in the area, stopping the dumping once and for all. The director of the mental health service, a female psychologist who still sees patients, spoke to me about the decision to make the change:

> We just changed the process for patient acceptance a year ago. What was happening was that we were having difficulty keeping up with our own referrals from our own primary care doctors. Access was extremely scarce. The only other clinic here is [inaudible], which is independent and has had financial difficulties. . . . They were cutting back their services and we were getting flooded with patients, and we could take care of all of them. . . . The other thing that was happening and it really made me angry was that we were also becoming the dumping ground for all patients of language from other places in the system, because we had made a commitment not to hire people without language capacity to serve our patient population more effectively, and then I'd be in fights with doctors in a nearby city, and the doctors would be saying, well, we're a primary care clinic, you have to take this patient. And I'm like, no, I don't and they're like, yes, I said you do because you're the only one with Spanish-speaking clinicians. And I said, you know what, I can appreciate that, but I think that you need to kick it up and take some leadership for the health care of your patients, because they are not going to respond to what your needs are, your patients, unless they're hearing it. So we were saying the same thing to Boston.

The director articulates the magnitude of her overcrowding problem and is flabbergasted by the sense of entitlement displayed by her sister clinic and Academic Medical Center 1, who demand she bow to their needs. She ultimately decided to close the unit to eliminate what she sees as a free rider problem that will not go away until others have an incentive to build their own capacity to treat patients from diverse cultural and linguistic communities. As she explains, "There's a part of me that feels like that if I take all of the people of color, the people with language in the whole system, then it doesn't force the system to respond to the needs of the patient, but ship them off."

The fight over patient dumping between hospitals within the same care network is strange in that Academic Medical Center 1 is the hub that connects all wheels in the system, and has in recent years invested large sums of money to fund the very systems of cultural and linguistically appropriate community-based services that allow these health centers to provide the quality of care they so vigorously extol and defend. These expenditures can be seen as a genuine effort to improve care in vulnerable communities while increasing the market for more intense and expensive care at Academic Medical Center 1.

The director of community services at Community Health Center quoted earlier told us that with contributions from Academic Medical Center 1 and other governmental and charitable organizations, they are financially secure and have vast resources to conduct myriad community and social services, including interpreter services in dozens of languages and a robust program of specialty refugee care and assistance. In her words, "It's never been hard to find funding, which is an amazing thing about this work. It's so well respected and presented in our system that whenever we've needed to expand there's always been ways to expand. In my last budget cycle it was $150,000 more than the previous year just because we needed it. New programs, new staff, and we got it."

According to the director, the hospital network's tax exempt status makes it easy to fund community-based programs, but she also has another theory about their willingness to fund programs like hers: a leadership determined to be the best in the world, even at providing culturally and linguistically sensitive community care. As she explained,

> I do think that there are champions who push it and I also think that the world is competitive. So, for example, there's a prestigious award that is given to the best hospital system, and Academic Medical Center 1 has applied for it years and years running and has never received it, and other hospitals have. And so one of the questions that community services pushed the hospital towards is to try and find out why these other hospitals are getting it and we're not. The big answer in that was this team came out and tried to show that what it is that they're doing is really they've incorporated community health work into the very fundamental mission of their hospital system. So, Academic Medical Center 1 is trying to learn from those. . . . There's been all these consultants who have come out to say how can we do it better and what is it that we need to be doing. So there is a desire to want to learn from other institutions that do it well and you know that's based on pure competition probably. [Laughs] Um, wanting to be the best. So, you know I think Academic Medical is seen as the best at many things but in this area there are probably people that are better.

The director appears to be enjoying the fruits of the hospital's investment in community care, yet continues to view their motives with skepticism. Her acknowledgement that other hospitals are still better reveals that, like the director of mental health at Community Health Center, she too feels they are shirking their responsibility in some ways by shifting the burden of cultural care onto to the satellite clinics instead of building their own capacity throughout the system. If they were to do so, fewer patients would be stuck in the emergency department because their inpatient unit might be larger, with full-time clinicians that speak languages other than English, and fewer patients would get dumped onto to satellite clinics still overwhelmed by demand from their own communities. But considering

America's commitment to a public-private system of health-care provision, they are still likely to be churned.

In this volume, we have argued that the culture of medicine itself, which includes the political economy of care, can complicate efforts to reduce racial, ethnic, or cultural disparities in care. This chapter illustrates how that process may occur. Regardless of bias or animus toward particular patients on the basis of their cultural or racial- or ethnic-based group membership, forces like finance and insurance and the structure and organization of the health-care system itself can limit the care that minorities receive.

One of the overarching critiques of current efforts to redress racial-ethnic disparities in care that we present in this volume is that these efforts focus too bluntly on broad cultural categories of group membership such as race and ethnicity as a way to improve equity in American health care. Other categories of cultural difference have meaning in this area as well, and a focus merely on race and ethnicity may not fully address these other axes of inequality—for example, by social class, by gender, by immigration status, or by more emergent forms of difference such as insurance status (free-care patient). This chapter reinforces the core message of the volume by focusing specifically on how structural forces in the way health care is organized and financed can also be a barrier to care for minority patients, and in a way that transcends—trumps—these older, broad notions of culture.

Notes

1. The notion of health care as a fundamental right is aggressively contested in America today, as evidenced by rise of the Tea Party movement and the vigorous battles in Congress and the courts over efforts to expand access to health insurance.

2. In April 2006, Massachusetts enacted a comprehensive health-care reform law, An Act Providing Access to Affordable, Quality, Accountable Health Care, commonly referred to as Chapter 58. The goal of the legislation was to move the state toward universal health insurance coverage through a series of reform measures. The measures included a requirement that almost all state residents have health insurance, as well as the creation of state-subsidized health insurance plans for low-income adults without access to other insurance. These subsidized plans are listed on a state-run insurance marketplace or exchange referred to as Commonwealth Connector (Pryor and Cohen 2009). Throughout this chapter, we use exchange, Commonwealth Connector, and Commonwealth Care interchangeably to denote any of the private plans available in the state-run marketplace. In March 2010, President Obama signed into law the Patient Protection and Affordable Care Act, also requiring nearly all U.S. residents to have health insurance and stabling a series of state-based health insurance marketplace or "exchanges" where individuals and small business can

purchase private health insurance plans that meet federal guidelines with the help of government subsidies.

3. We use generic names to describe clinics and hospitals where we conducted research to mask their identity. This chapter examines the relationship between two units in a large elite academic medical center in Boston and one of its own community health-care centers outside of town.

4. *Free care* is the colloquial term for the Uncompensated Care Pool set up by the State of Massachusetts to provide health care for residents who are not eligible for public or private health insurance or cannot afford it. The free care system identified (and disproportionately supported with higher reimbursement rates) two institutions for the care of the poor and indigent: Cambridge Health Alliance and Boston Medical Center, the "safety net hospitals." Boston Medical Center does not have a psychiatric inpatient department, so any psychiatric emergency room in the Boston area needing to place a patient in inpatient care would only have one choice for free care referral, Cambridge Health Alliance, which is regularly filled with referrals from within their own network of feeder hospitals and clinics. On October 1, 2007, the Health Safety Net replaced the Uncompensated Care Pool. To be covered by the Health Safety Net, Massachusetts residents must be uninsured or underinsured and have no access to affordable health coverage. People of any income with large medical bills that they cannot pay are also eligible. Citizenship or immigration status does not affect eligibility. The Health Safety Net pays all or some of the medically necessary services at Massachusetts community health centers and hospitals, depending on age and income. To be covered, services must be on the Mass Health Standard list of covered services.

5. The importance of community health center was recognized by the Affordable Care Act, which included an $11 billion investment in the expansion of community health centers across the country. This investment is expected to make affordable, cost-effective, high-quality preventive and primary care services available to nearly twice as many people regardless of their insurance status or ability to pay (see http://www.healthcare.gov).

References

Brandon, William P., Rajeshwari Sundaram, and Ashley A. Dunham. 2009. "Multiple Switching in Medicaid Managed Care: A Proportional Hazards Model." *Journal of Health Care for the Poor and Underserved* 20(4): 1124–141.

Cunningham, Peter J., Gloria J. Bazzoli, and Aaron Katz. 2008. "Caught in the Competitive Crossfire: Safety Net Providers Balance Margin and Mission in a Profit Driven Health Care Market." *Health Affairs* 27(5): w374–82.

Dorn, Stan, Ian Hill, and Sara Hogan. 2009. "The Secrets of Massachusetts' Success: Why 97 Percent of State Residents Have Health Coverage." A report prepared by the State Health Access Reform Evaluation. Washington, D. C.: Robert Wood Johnson Foundation.

Grogan, Colleen M., and Michael K. Gusmano. 2009. "Political Strategies of Safety-Net Providers in Response to Medicaid Managed Care Reforms." *Journal of Health Politics, Policy and Law* 34(1): 5–35.

Hunt, James W. 2005. "Community Health Centers' Impact on the Political and Economic Environment: the Massachusetts Example." *Journal of Ambulatory Care Management* 28(4): 340–47.

Hunter, Mary-Lyons, and Lawrence Taeseng Park. 2010. "Gateway Communities: Providing Healthcare, Negotiating Citizenship for New Immigrant Populations." Unpublished manuscript.

Long, Sharon K., and Karen Stockley. 2010. "Sustaining Health Reform in a Recession: An Update on Massachusetts as of Fall 2009." *Health Affairs* 29(6): 1234–241.

Massachusetts Division of Health Care Finance and Policy. 2010. "Health Insurance Coverage in Massachusetts: Results from the 2008–2010 Massachusetts Health Insurance Surveys. Boston: Massachusetts Department of Health and Human Services.

Parmet, Wendy. 2009. "Litigation Amidst Reform: The Boston Medical Center Case." *New England Journal of Medicine* 361(19): 1819–821.

Pryor, Carol, and Andrew Cohen. 2009. "Consumers' Experience in Massachusetts: Lessons for National Health Reform." Menlo Park, Calif.: The Henry J. Kaiser Family Foundation.

Rhodes, Lorna. 1991. *Emptying Beds: The Work of an Emergency Psychiatric Unit.* Berkeley: University of California Press.

Weismann, Joel S., and Judy Ann Bigby. 2009. "Massachusetts Health Care Reform—Near Universal Coverage at What Cost?" *New England Journal of Medicine* 361(21): 2012–15.

Index

Boldface numbers refer to figures and tables.